TURN UP
YOUR
FAT BURN!™

TURN UP
YOUR
FAT BURN!™

Go from *frustrated to fit* with our
REVOLUTIONARY
4-week **weight-loss** program

ALYSSA SHAFFER
and the editors of **Prevention**® magazine

RODALE.

© 2011 by Rodale Inc.

Photographs © 2011 by Rodale Inc.

All rights reserved. No part of this publication may be reproduced or transmitted in any form or by any means, electronic or mechanical, including photocopying, recording, or any other information storage and retrieval system, without the written permission of the publisher.

Prevention and Turn Up Your Fat Burn are registered trademarks of Rodale Inc.

Printed in the United States of America

Rodale Inc. makes every effort to use acid-free ∞, recycled paper ♺.

Book design by Carol Angstadt

Photographs by Mitch Mandel/Rodale Inc.

Library of Congress Cataloging-in-Publication Data

Shaffer, Alyssa.
  Turn up your fat burn : go from frustrated to fit with our revolutionary 4-week weight-loss program! / Alyssa Shaffer and the editors of Prevention magazine.
      p.   cm.
  Includes bibliographical references and index.
  ISBN 978–1–60961–031–9 hardcover
  1. Weight loss—Popular works.   2. Reducing exercises—Popular works.   I. Title.
RM222.2.S463   2011
613.2′5—dc22   2011001991

2   4   6   8   10   9   7   5   3   1   hardcover

We inspire and enable people to improve their lives and the world around them.

For more of our products visit prevention.com/shop or call 800-848-4735.

To Scott, Layla, and Nolan:
You make every day sunny and bright.

Contents

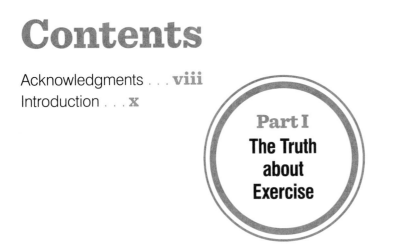

Part I
The Truth about Exercise

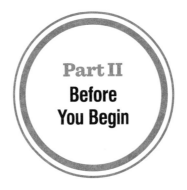

Part II
Before You Begin

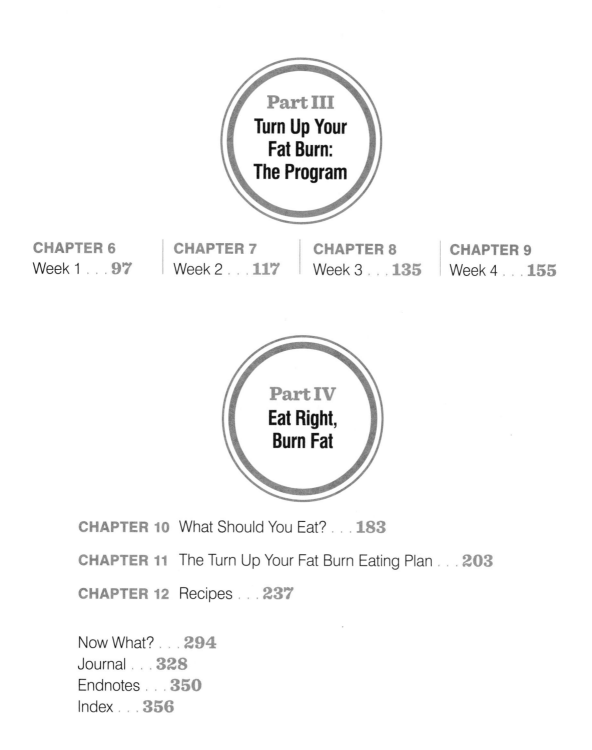

Part III
Turn Up Your Fat Burn: The Program

Part IV
Eat Right, Burn Fat

Acknowledgments

Although much of writing is a solitary effort, this book would not have been possible without the help of a great many people. I'm deeply grateful to everyone involved for their hard work, support, contributions, assistance, and valuable feedback.

To Fabio Comana, who helped me turn a seed into a flowering plan. Your patience and guidance were invaluable, and your knowledge and understanding of all things fitness help countless individuals live longer, stronger, and healthier lives.

To the Turn Up Your Fat Burn test panel: Marixsa Ali, Pete Brown, Annette Carpien, Kathy Chartier, Burt Duren, Pam Garin, Laura Goldy, Kimberly Hampsey, Anne Jenkins, Leslie Kingston, Wendy Klemka, Pat Lisetski, Loretta Mariscano, Susan Mauser, Lisa Miller, Patricia Rizzotto, Joyce Salter, Catherine Schaper, Audrey Stasak, Leslie Tang, Hans Wagner, Cindy Wenrich, and Michael Wunderly. Thank you so much for your perseverance, humor, and dedication and for your continued efforts to stay fit. Your efforts were impressive and inspirational.

To my editor, Andrea Au Levitt, without whose support and guidance this project would never have been possible. Thank you for believing in me and in the Turn Up Your Fat Burn plan. To Marielle Messing, for her amazing organization and assistance in putting together the test panel program and helping to guide it along. To Budd Coates and Tammy Strunk at the Rodale Energy Center, for helping determine those all-important VT1s and putting the plan in action. To Tracy Gensler, who developed the scrumptious and satisfying meal plan and contributed the cutting-edge nutrition research. To Michele Stanten, for her support, enthusiasm, and valuable feedback. And to the super-efficient and impressive photo and design team of Carol Angstadt, Mitch Mandel, Susan Eugster, and Anne Marie Amatulli: The images on these pages are a testament to your talent!

The greatest thanks goes to my family and friends: To my wonderful husband, Scott, who after more than 22 years keeps me strong and centered, and to my amazing children, Nolan and Layla, who inspire me with their wonder, patience, and love. To Terry Manzella, who's always there whenever I need her with invaluable assistance and support. To my training partners, Elaine Yu, Judy Marshall, and Robin Durawa for their encouragement and feedback even when we're on that third bike loop around the park or 4 miles into a run. To Gail Shust and Avery Brandon, whose monthly dinners help keep me sane. And to Dad, Susan, Andy, Jill, Cynthia, Joel, Lauren, and Jay, for all their love and confidence.

Introduction

As a writer and the former fitness director of a major health and fitness magazine, I've done the old "rev up your metabolism" or "drop a dress size in just a few weeks" story at least a hundred times.

I've written about running, walking, skating, hiking, swimming, belly dancing, jazzercise, circus arts, beach-body boot camp, kickboxing, and pretty much any other type of cardiovascular workout you can think of that will raise your heart rate and get you sweating. I've described at least a thousand ways to strengthen your abs, your arms, your butt, your thighs, and any other muscle group you might want to tone, buff, sculpt, or lift. I've investigated some pretty wacky diet recommendations and even explored how your clothes can help you burn more calories (the theory: the more comfortable you are, the more you'll move around, the bigger your burn). I've interviewed top researchers from universities from every corner of the globe, spent untold hours online looking up research studies, and called upon literally hundreds of trainers, from Hollywood types who work with some of the biggest celebrities in movies, TV, and music to your average Joes and Janes who teach at the local YMCA.

So I didn't expect to hear anything all that new or different when I picked up the phone to call Fabio Comana, an exercise physiologist with the American Council on Exercise (ACE), while researching an article about different ways to lose fat and boost metabolism. For some time, I've known that he's always up to date on the latest research and theories about exercise and performance. He also knows virtually everything about what works and what doesn't when it comes to helping the average person get results.

His organization, ACE, is also fabulous. They bill themselves as "America's Authority on Fitness" and don't disappoint. This nonprofit group is committed to promoting safe, effective exercise and physical activity. They sponsor cutting-edge research into all sorts of fitness products and claims (among the many devices they've debunked over the years are toning shoes, oxygenated water, and electronic muscle stimulation machines). Moreover, they are one of the largest independent fitness certification, education, and training groups in the world, with more than 50,000 certified professionals (including yours truly). Fabio is one of their go-to spokespersons for the media, as well as a faculty member at San Diego State University and the University of California, San Diego—he really knows his stuff.

I knew Fabio would provide some good ideas for my article, though I didn't expect anything groundbreaking to come out of our interview. But when Fabio started explaining his theories about how to help the average person burn more fat and boost his or her metabolism, I sat up and listened. His ideas were not only steeped in science but completely different from anything I'd heard before. I was typing as quickly as I could (which, after my 20 years as a journalist, is pretty darn fast) and couldn't get my questions out fast enough. I knew, then and there, that this was the basis for a program that would truly make a major difference in the way people think about exercise.

Fabio outlined two new approaches to exercise. Individually, each sounds like an amazingly effective way to work out. Together, they are a one-two punch, a revolutionary program that provides results like nothing you've ever seen before.

The first new approach is called metabolic circuit training. It boosts metabolism by building lean muscle through a nonstop strength routine that will keep you burning calories even hours after you've finished. The second is a unique cardio regimen called VT training that's designed to turn your body into a more efficient fat-burning machine. Both ideas have been studied extensively by exercise scientists as ways to help the average person lose weight, burn fat, and get fit. In a few small ways, similar concepts have made their way to fitness centers and gyms around the country. This is the first full, real-world application of either approach—let alone both!

I was so excited about Fabio's concept that I asked him to work with me on a program that would help ordinary people who have been frustrated with their weight-loss efforts achieve the results they really want. And he agreed!

We decided on a few rules about the program. It couldn't require a lot of time or equipment. It couldn't be superhard but had to be challenging enough to get results. And, of course, it needed to be a plan that people could realistically continue to follow for lasting results.

We recruited a panel of nearly two dozen ordinary men and women—teachers, business executives, retirees, husbands and wives, and sisters. Many had tried virtually every popular diet over the past 2 decades and were in a perpetual cycle of losing and gaining weight. Others had watched the pounds stealthily creep on each year. Some were just plain frustrated that despite their current exercise routines, they couldn't seem to lose any extra pounds.

We asked these 23 men and women to try our plan for 4 weeks while following a healthy eating plan. Their results were truly astounding. On average, they lost nearly 7 pounds and 3 inches while cutting nearly 1.5 percent body fat; our biggest loser dropped 22$\frac{1}{2}$ pounds! They accomplished all that by exercising just 4 days a week for an average of 35 minutes each time. Moreover, they all reported more energy and body confidence. And they were excited about what the future held, now that they knew how to maximize their fat burn and get the most out of every minute of exercise. You'll find out more about their experiences throughout the book.

But before we dive into the details of the plan, you're going to learn how and why it works. Understanding the science behind the Turn Up Your Fat Burn program will help you stick with it so you get the results you really want.

Alyssa Shaffer

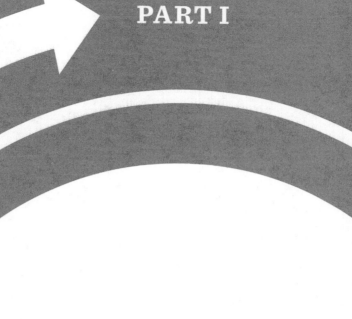

The Truth about Exercise

CHAPTER 1

Understanding Fat So You Can Burn More of It

All of us—even the skinniest supermodel and the leanest ultramarathoner—have body fat. You can't survive without it. Fat (aka adipose tissue) stores energy for when you really need it. It cushions your organs, helps regulate your body temperature, and produces some important hormones that help control your hunger and appetite. It's just that most of us carry around a little—or a lot—more fat than we'd like or than is good for us.

THE FACTS ABOUT FAT

Among American women, an average of 31 percent of total body weight is fat; for men, the number is about 24 percent.[1] Most adipose (fat) tissue is located under the skin (subcutaneous fat) and around the internal organs (visceral fat), as well as in bone marrow and breasts. Visceral fat, the kind you often can't see, is a deep fat that's particularly dangerous, especially in the abdominal area. It increases the risk of high cholesterol and impaired liver function, as well as of heart disease, diabetes, insulin resistance, and other health problems.

The good news is that visceral fat responds fairly well to exercise. Researchers from Duke University, for example, found that participants in their study who exercised vigorously dropped about 8 percent of their visceral fat in 6 months, while those who did nothing actually gained about 9 percent more visceral fat.[2]

This deep-belly fat is also linked to high levels of stress. In response to chronic stress, the body creates more of the hormone cortisol, which is known to trigger the storage of visceral fat. Since exercise is also a great way to bust stress, it's a double weapon against this dangerous type of body fat.

Subcutaneous fat is the kind that gives us curves, but for plenty of people, it's hanging around in excess, especially in the trunk, the backs of the arms, the top of the back, and around the butt and thighs. While it's not as dangerous as visceral fat, too much subcutaneous fat can be unhealthy, especially when it raises your body mass index (BMI) above 25. (BMI is a measurement of body fat based on weight and height. A "normal" weight falls within 18.5 to 24.9, while 25 to 29.9 is considered "overweight," and 30 or more is considered obese.)

Just like you can't live without any body fat, you also need the fat in food to survive. Dietary fat carries vital vitamins like A, D, E, and K, as well as other important chemical substances. Fat also helps create and maintain cellular membranes, and it keeps your skin and nails strong and healthy. Fat can come from plant or animal sources and is energy dense—it has more than twice as many calories (9 per gram) as protein or carbs (4 per gram each).

There's a whole group of dietary fats, but chemically, most fats are triglycerides. While body fat is also composed primarily of triglycerides, all the foods that you consume—carbohydrates, fat, and protein—will eventually be stored as fat tissue if you eat too much of them. It's a complicated process, but basically, the calories you don't burn off over a certain period of time are converted into triglycerides and are then transported to fat cells, where they are stored for future use. This is great if you're worried about famine. It's not so great in this day and age, when the closest hamburger is a dollar meal away.

HOW EXERCISE BURNS FAT

Now that we have some of the science of fat straight, let's look at how exercise helps you get rid of unwanted body fat.

When your body needs fuel during exercise, triglycerides are freed from the fat cells and broken down into fatty acids. A complex metabolic process turns the fatty acids into adenosine triphosphate (ATP), a compound that is the body's primary energy source.

When a muscle fiber contracts, the energy to move it comes from ATP. Only a limited amount of ATP is stored in the muscles, so your body has to make more of it to keep on working. ATP is produced through chemical reactions that are aerobic (requiring oxygen), anaerobic (oxygen not needed), or facilitated by a compound called creatine phosphate.

Your body's primary, go-to fuel source is glucose (stored carbs), which it readily turns into ATP. But your muscles actually prefer burning fat for fuel, since fat is relatively easy to extract and provides a comparatively large amount of energy. (*Note:* Your body will always burn some amount of carbs and fat together, but the ratio of how much carbs versus fat shifts as the intensity of your workout increases.) You'll typically burn fat stored in muscle tissue (muscle triglycerides) before you burn the fat stored in adipose tissue (what we think of as body fat). It usually takes at least 10 minutes of exercise for the body to start drawing from body fat stores. Your body can also break down proteins for energy, but that takes more effort, so it generally won't go there unless absolutely necessary. Of course, diet also plays an important role in which fuel is utilized, so following a well-balanced diet that is relatively low in fat has a great impact.

When you're at rest (sleeping, sitting at your desk, channel surfing on the couch), your body generally relies on both fatty acids and glucose for fuel, at a rate of about 1 calorie per minute. According to the American Council on Exercise, about 50 percent of this resting calorie burn can come from fatty acids. In a fit individual, however, as much as 70 percent of resting calories can come from fatty acids.[3] The better shape you're in, the more fat you'll burn all day long, even when you're just hanging out.

When you start to move around—when you exercise—your heart and lungs have to get oxygen into your muscles in order to produce ATP. (Most cardiovascular exercises are called aerobic, which literally translates to "with oxygen.") As we'll discuss in more detail later, when you're exercising or moving about with relatively low effort, most of the fuel needed to charge your muscles will come from fat, although some carbs are always used at the same time. (There's an expression among exercise physiologists that "fat burns in a carbohydrate flame," meaning that fat oxidation always takes place along with the breakdown of some carbs.) That's because burning fat takes more oxygen than burning glucose. During low-intensity exercise, oxygen is more readily available, so fats are used more often as a fuel source. As exercise intensity increases, the percentage of carbs burned becomes higher.

If you keep increasing intensity, eventually your cardiovascular system can't get enough oxygen into the cells fast enough to produce ATP. How soon you reach this point depends on your genetic makeup and how much training you do. The better shape you're in, the longer you'll be able to keep burning fat as exercise intensity increases. From then on, the only way you can keep those ATP supplies coming is through an anaerobic ("without oxygen") process. Your body can't keep up this intensity for very long. With anaerobic metabolism, your body primarily uses glucose to create ATP. (You can also get fuel from creatine phosphate, but only in limited amounts.) After that, you bonk.

Why exercise when I can diet?

There's no arguing with the basic weight-loss equation: In order to drop excess pounds, you need to burn more calories than you consume. You can do this by drastically cutting calories, but for many of us, dieting alone is simply too hard. To lose just a pound a week, you'd need to cut 3,500 calories from your diet, or 500 fewer calories a day than you are used to eating. While you can keep this up for a few days or even a few weeks, eventually it becomes just too difficult to keep slashing calories.

That's where exercise comes in. Scientific journals are filled with evidence that regular physical activity not only will help you lose weight (and live longer) but is crucial to staying leaner. The American College of Sports Medicine even created an official recommendation that anyone who wants to lose weight should try to create a deficit of 500 to 1,000 calories a day through a combination of diet and physical activity.[6] Among participants in the renowned National Weight Control Registry (the largest ongoing study of successful long-term weight loss, consisting of more than 5,000 individuals who have lost at least 30 pounds and kept that weight off for at least 1 year), consistent exercise is the single best predictor of long-term weight maintenance.[7]

Think of it this way: If you add 60 minutes of activity a day, even just a brisk walk, you'll burn another 2,300 calories a week. Over a year, that's about 35 pounds you've either kept off or lost.

Bottom line: If you're in this for the long haul, dieting alone can be tough. To get the best results, you also need to exercise.

And yet . . .

Sometimes no matter how many miles you walk on the treadmill or pedal away on the bike or elliptical, you can still feel very frustrated when you step on the scale or look in the mirror. While exercise is undeniably good for your heart, lungs, and brain, it can be bad for your psyche if you're not getting the positive results you want.

WHAT AM I DOING WRONG?

Let's start with what you're doing *right*. You don't need a PhD in exercise physiology to know that any form of physical activity will improve your health. Every time you raise your heart rate with aerobic exercise, you're helping your heart and lungs get stronger and more efficient. You're bathing your brain in feel-good hormones; you're pushing oxygenated blood throughout your body to deliver important nutrients to your tissues; you're helping your body get a better night's sleep; you're even helping to spark your sex life. When you add strength and flexibility training to the mix, you're also building stronger bones; revving your metabolism; and keeping your joints, ligaments, tendons, and muscles limber throughout the decades of your life.

Yet many of us don't see the weight-loss results we expect because of how much, how often, and how hard we're exercising. Take a look at these common workout mistakes—some may sound pretty familiar.

Mistake #1: You're caught in an exercise rut.

When you do the same activity day after day, week after week, your mind isn't the only thing that gets bored—your muscles do, too. Whether you take the same daily 30-minute walk around the neighborhood loop or do a few sets of the same old strength moves, after a while your body stops being challenged and your results plateau.

Mend it: Change things up. Go for a hike on the weekend instead of doing your usual power walk. Find new strength moves that work the same muscles. (There are some great ones in the following chapters.) Try a new type of exercise by slipping in a workout DVD. Any little way to mix things up and challenge yourself with something new is a step in the right direction.

Mistake #2: You're loyal to cardio.

I have friends who run, bike, or swim religiously but can't get rid of stubborn fat around their tummies, hips, and thighs. It's because they haven't picked up a pair of weights in years. While aerobic exercise is good for your body and soul, if you don't balance those workouts with some strength exercises, you're not only compromising your results but missing a key component of health and fitness. Resistance training—lifting weights or strength training—is the only way to increase lean muscle mass. That's important on many levels, especially as we start to get older.

Beginning in their thirties, women begin to lose about $\frac{1}{2}$ pound of muscle per year. (Men usually hold on to muscle longer, but the rate of muscle loss speeds up dramatically after age 60.) Since muscle burns through calories even at rest, losing it will noticeably slow metabolism. This is one big reason many of us see that "middle-age spread" beginning in our forties.

A study from Skidmore College found that exercisers who combined cardio with a high-intensity, total-body resistance routine lost more than twice as much body fat—including twice as much belly fat—over 12 weeks than those who followed a moderate-intensity cardio plan.[8] (You'll find out more about the many benefits of strength training later in this book.)

Mend it: Substitute a couple of strength sessions for cardio days. On our plan, you'll be lifting weights twice a week, hitting all of your body's major muscle groups.

Mistake #3: You're stuck in a "fat-burning" zone.

If you hop aboard a treadmill, elliptical trainer, stairclimber, or other cardio machine at the gym, you may see a programming option that allows you to stay in a "fat-burning" zone. It's based on the fact that at lower intensities, the body uses a greater percentage of its fat stores for fuel. Sounds great! You don't have to work as hard *and* you're sucking some of that fat out of your belly, butt, and thighs.

But do the math and you'll see the problem. At a lower intensity level, your body will indeed burn a higher percentage of fat than carbs but still burn fewer calories overall.

Here's an example. A 150-pound woman who walks on a treadmill at 3 mph (a 20-minute mile) burns about 112 calories in 30 minutes. At this moderate intensity, she burns about half of those calories from fat, or about 56 fat calories. If she were to take that workout into a brisk walk for 30 minutes at 4 mph (a 15-minute mile), only about 40 percent of her calorie burn might be from fat. But she'd be burning more calories over-all—about 170 in those 30 minutes, or about 68 calories from fat.

Mend it: In the next chapter, you'll learn how to burn more calories and make more of those calories come from fat. You will increase your overall effort by doing intervals—periods of higher intensity followed by a slower recovery pace.

If you're already exercising regularly, the Turn Up Your Fat Burn program is designed to help you get past some of these common mistakes and achieve the fitness and fat-loss results you want. And if you're not involved in an exercise program right now, there's no better time to start.

SO HOW DO I BURN MORE FAT?

All of this brings us back to the reason you probably picked this book up in the first place: to learn how to burn more fat and lose more weight when you exercise.

Here's where things start to get really interesting. Most of the time when you plan a workout, you're focusing on two goals: how long you should go and how hard you should work. We've seen that at a low intensity, you burn a greater percentage of calories from fat, and at a higher intensity, you burn more calories. What if you could burn more calories overall *and* more of them from fat? In other words, how can you train your body to tap into those body-fat stores easier and faster and become a more efficient fat-burning machine?

The secret is a metabolic marker called the Ventilatory Threshold 1 or VT1. This sounds complicated, but it's not. Honest! VT1 is the point

1. You deliver more oxygen to your muscles. The more oxygen your muscles get, the more efficiently your cells will burn (oxidize) fat.

2. Your muscle and fat cells become more sensitive to the hormone epinephrine, which makes it easier to release fatty acids into the bloodstream.

3. You improve your circulation, which means faster delivery of fatty acids to the muscles to be used as fuel. You also boost the specialized protein transporters that move fatty acids into the muscle cells so that fat becomes more readily available.

4. You increase the amount of fatty acids that enter a muscle, which means you'll be able to burn even more fat.

5. You increase the number and size of mitochondria (the body's "fat-burning engines") in muscle cells.

6. You increase the number of enzymes that help speed up or break down fatty acid molecules.

during exercise when you shift from burning fat as your primary fuel to burning more carbs. Just before VT1, you're burning 51 percent fat, 49 percent carbs. The ratio then shifts, first to an even level, and then to 51 percent carbs, 49 percent fat. After the VT1 point, the ratio starts to shift more quickly, and you burn carbs at a much faster level.

Sounds a little bit like the old fat-burning zone so far, right? But as you just learned, the problem with sticking to the fat-burning zone is that overall calorie burn is too low. With VT training, your goal is to raise your VT1 level so that you'll burn more calories overall and at the higher fat-to-carb ratio, which ultimately will help you lose weight more quickly.

How can you raise your VT1 level? Intervals. When you work out, you should alternate between a slightly higher intensity (briefly pushing your body to work just a bit beyond VT1) and a recovery period at a slightly lower intensity (staying at VT1 so that you are burning as much fat as possible). This will allow you to raise your overall VT1 levels after just a few weeks of training. (In Chapter 5, you'll learn how to determine your VT1, your personal fat-burning point.)

One study found that after a few months of training at and above VT1, subjects were able to shift their VT1 levels (and therefore burn more calories) by an average of 15 percent.[10] That means a workout that used to burn 300 calories now burns 345! Another study found that women who exercised three times a week for an hour just above VT1 started to see a slight reduction in weight and BMI after just 2 weeks and a 6.2 percent difference in BMI after 8 weeks.[11]

The more you train at and just above VT1, the more efficiently you'll burn fat. You'll not only be burning more calories during your workout, but you'll be drawing a higher percentage of those calories from your body-fat stores. This more effective workout will help you get the fat-loss results you really want. In fact, the better shape you're in, the harder you can work (and the more calories you'll torch) while still burning mostly fat.

Best of all, when you teach your body to burn fat more efficiently, it starts to do that all day long—even when you're just hanging out. The

VT1 versus VT2

In this book, when we refer to Ventilatory Threshold (VT) training, we're talking about raising your VT1 level, which is the point at which your body shifts from burning mostly fat to mostly carbs. There's also a VT2 level, which is the point at which lactate and its by-products rapidly increase in your blood. You might hear some athletes refer to this as the lactate threshold.

VT2 is the highest level of activity you can sustain (in well-trained individuals, it's about 30 to 60 minutes). At this point, you'll really "feel the burn"; that burning sensation is caused by the lactic acid and its by-products. But don't worry, you won't be seeing much of VT2 training until your final week, when it's used as an extra challenge. The Turn Up Your Fat Burn plan concentrates mostly on VT1 training to increase your fat-burning metabolism.

average person burns only 4 to 6 percent of his or her **weekly calorie** intake through exercise, assuming three weekly sessions **of 20 min-** utes each. But when the average man increases his VT1 **level by as lit-** tle as 10 percent, he'll burn 263 more calories daily—a **pound of fat** every 2 weeks, without even counting the workouts. **The average** woman will burn 178 more calories, which means an **extra pound** about every 3 weeks.

Lift weights, burn fat

Most of us think of cardio as the only way to burn body **fat. There's no** arguing that you will reduce the most body fat if you incorporate aero- bic training into your exercise routine. But resistance **training also** plays an important role in burning fat.

There's a long list of benefits of strength training: **helping build** stronger bones, reducing blood pressure, lowering LDL ("bad") choles- terol, elevating HDL ("good") cholesterol, improving heart health, and even reducing the risks of diabetes and arthritis. But it's **in the area of** weight loss and weight maintenance that resistance **training might** have the biggest effect. Muscle plays a very important **role in metabo-** lism, or how your body burns calories. Muscle is more **metabolically** active than fat. Even at rest, muscle burns about twice **the calories** that fat does—roughly 7 to 10 calories for a pound of muscle, **compared** with 2 or 3 calories for a pound of fat.[12] So the more **muscle you have,** the more calories you'll burn all day long. Just how **much people** increase their metabolism by strength training is **debated among** exercise physiologists, but there is evidence that **regular strength** training can increase resting metabolism by 10 percent (that's the amount of calories burned to maintain basic body **functions, not** including exercise, eating, and other activities).[13] The **average person** burns about 2,000 calories a day, 60 to 75 percent while **at rest. That's** 1,200 to 1,500 calories a day. Boost resting metabolism **by 10 percent,** and you'll burn an extra 120 to 150 calories a day. That's **another pound** you're keeping off every 23 days just by getting in shape **and building a** little muscle.

Adding resistance training is especially important when you're trying to lose weight. Dieting alone will shift the numbers on the scale, but you'll be losing lean muscle mass along with fat. When you add weight training, you'll preserve and even build your muscle tissue while still getting rid of the fat. Think of it this way: For each pound you lose while dieting and *not* exercising, $^3/_4$ pound will come from fat mass and $^1/_4$ pound will come from muscle. When you diet and add strength exercise, you lose a full pound of fat while gaining an extra $^1/_4$ pound of calorie-burning muscle.

Research backs this point: A study from the University of Alabama at Birmingham found that among women who lost more than 25 pounds, those who did resistance training were able to keep that muscle mass, while those who just did cardio or no exercise at all lost lean muscle. They showed a significantly lower resting metabolism, which means their metabolism dropped along with the pounds they lost, while the strength-training group kept their metabolism elevated.[14] Research also shows that a diet-only program can lower resting metabolism by as much as 20 percent (which means you'll burn about 300 fewer calories each day).[15]

Then there's the amount of fat you can burn during resistance training itself. Cardio is still queen when it comes to drawing on your fat stores, especially when you're exercising at or around VT1. But research shows that the body will also use fat both during and after resistance training. A 2007 study published in the *Journal of Applied Physiology* found that men who did a strength workout had a 78 percent increase in glycerol levels (a marker for fat burning in the body) during exercise and a 75 percent increase after training, compared with a day they did no exercise. Fat burning was 105 percent higher on workout day than on rest day.[16]

That difference can translate into some very real changes in your body composition. One study found that women and men who did only cardio exercise lost 4 pounds but gained no muscle over an 8-week period; those who cut out half the cardio but added strength training lost 10 pounds of fat and added 2 pounds of muscle.[17] Another study found that people who did resistance training along with cardio lost 44 percent more fat than those who lost weight by diet alone.[18]

The Turn Up Your Fat Burn program is designed to maximize your fat-burning ability by bringing together these two fitness fundamentals: an aerobic conditioning program that will elevate your VT1 level so you burn more fat with each workout and a strength routine that will boost your metabolism and keep you burning more fat all day long. Of course, the idea of doing both strength and cardio isn't new. But the key to getting results and helping you lose that extra fat lies in the way the workouts themselves are designed.

LESLIE KINGSTON

Age: 52

Height: 5'10"

Pounds lost: 11

Inches lost: $8\frac{1}{4}$

What she's most proud of:
"I've started to accomplish what I set out to do—losing weight and getting back into a regular exercise routine. And I lost double digits in 1 month!"

Favorite Foods: Peanut butter and honey on Wasa crackers; tuna on popcorn cakes; edamame

A veteran of many diet and fitness plans, Leslie Kingston was skeptical when she first looked over the Turn Up Your Fat Burn routine. "I've worked out in the past, but usually for an hour a day, 6 days a week, and I'd never been able to be on a diet without feeling like I was starving! I figured there was no way I'd see results exercising just 30 to 45 minutes a few days a week and eating this amount of food."

But after 4 weeks on the program, Leslie is a believer. "I followed the plan exactly as instructed, and I am absolutely amazed at the results." At her final weigh-in, Leslie had dropped almost 11 pounds and lost almost 3 inches from her waistline, $2\frac{1}{2}$ inches from her hips, and $\frac{3}{4}$ inch from her thighs.

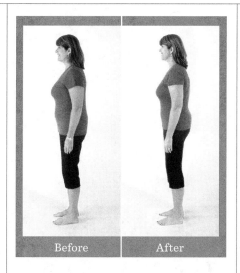

Before   After

"I had to go to a black-tie event, and I pulled out a dress from my closet that was a full size smaller than what I usually wore. I put it on, and it looked amazing!" She also reports that her once-tight jeans feel roomier, her arms are more defined, and her belly looks flatter. But her favorite benefit of all may be the improvement in her golf game. "I think the exercises have made a difference in my core strength, balance, and flexibility. My handicap actually went down two strokes in 1 month!"

Leslie felt she needed a change after looking through some photos taken at her youngest son's college graduation, when she weighed upward of 196 pounds. "I felt pretty good about myself until I saw those pictures. I was shocked to see what I'd become."

She says the variety of the program—an ever-changing mix of strength moves and cardio intervals—kept her involved and on track. "Every workout I'd done before was just more of the same: more reps, more weights, more time. Mixing it up kept me motivated to continue." Her favorite part of all the workouts: doing the sprints in the Week 4 cardio routine. "I loved being able to push myself for a short time, then take a break and do it again. It was a great challenge but really fulfilling to finish it!"

Challenges of her own came up over the month on the panel—she was stuck on an island in the Caribbean during a hurricane and had to cope with the news of a terminally ill sibling. But she says sticking to the plan helped her get through it all. "I actually was looking forward to getting up at 5:45 a.m. to get on the treadmill."

As a pescatarian (she eats fish but not chicken or other kinds of meat), Leslie says it was easy enough to stick to a healthy eating plan. "I don't cook, and I don't like to count calories, but I was able to figure out my portion sizes pretty easily, get in more fruits and veggies, and finish the day feeling totally satisfied."

Nowadays she's looking through her photos with much more satisfaction but says she's not done yet. "I can't wait to get back into some of those cocktail dresses that I couldn't zip up anymore," she says. "I'm back into a routine that is manageable and works for me, and I'm on the fitness wagon for good!"

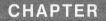

CHAPTER 2

Making the Science Work for You

Now that we've sold you on the whys of the Turn Up Your Fat Burn plan's unique strength and cardio combo, let's get into more detail on the hows.

MAXIMIZING YOUR METABOLISM

Most strength workouts are designed to build lean muscle; they ultimately increase your metabolism but don't *maximize* your metabolism. That takes more than basic dumbbell biceps curls or triceps presses followed by some rest time, a trip to the water fountain, and a chat with a friend.

Our metabolic strength workouts are designed to help you turn up your fat burn by working several different muscle groups at the same time or close together, minimizing the amount of rest between exercises. You move in a circuit from one exercise to the next, taking only the time you need to find the right weight and get yourself into a starting position. After you complete all the exercises once through, you take a brief rest and then do them all again. Then, during Weeks 2, 3, and 4, you have the option of doing the circuit a third and final time.

By the end of the strength session, you've fully worked all of your major muscles and even had a bit of a cardio workout. This type of training can be a bit intense if you're not used to it, but once you get the hang of it, you'll really feel the difference.

Metabolic circuit workouts are effective for several reasons.

You burn more calories.

In a typical strength routine in which you focus on one muscle at a time for several sets, then take time between sets to allow the muscles to recover, the calorie burn is relatively low. According to the *Compendium of Physical Activity*, a go-to guide for exercise physiologists, a standard strength routine has about 5 to 6 METs (metabolic equivalents).[19] One MET is the amount of energy a body uses at rest, or about 1 to 1.5 calories a minute, so you'll burn about 7 calories a minute.

A circuit workout has almost 8 METs—about 9 to 10 calories a minute.[20] That means you'll burn 25 percent more calories just by doing a circuit workout instead of an ordinary strength routine. And the total doesn't even count the calories burned in the anaerobic (without oxygen) phase that occurs during the strength repetitions, which means the actual number of calories can be notably higher. Researchers from the University of Southern Maine found that significantly more energy is burned during this anaerobic phase than scientists once thought.[21]

You work your heart and lungs along with your muscles.

Most strength workouts are strictly anaerobic. The body burns carbs to fuel the short bursts of intensity required to lift and lower the weight to fatigue. In circuit training, your heart rate stays elevated during the period of lower intensity when you move from one exercise to the next, which makes the routine significantly more aerobic. That's key, because the only time you're burning fat is when you're doing aerobic exercise. In just a half hour, you'll be doing a workout that's the caloric equivalent of walking or jogging a 12-minute mile—but with the added strength gains.

And since the Turn Up Your Fat Burn plan includes cardio workouts on the VT1 interval days (we'll get to that in a minute), the combined benefits are exponential. In fact, one study from Ball State University found that women who did both resistance and aerobic training had significantly higher fitness gains in both strength and cardiovascular conditioning than those who did only aerobic activity.[22]

You get a bigger "afterburn."

Exercise isn't the only time your body burns more calories. After the workout is over, your body's furnace stays stoked as it works to get back to its natural resting state. This process is known as EPOC, or excess postoxygen consumption. Right after exercise is when the biggest changes happen. Your heart rate is still slightly elevated, and your body has to work to repay all the efforts made during exercise itself. And your metabolism can remain elevated for up to 38 hours through the latter phase of EPOC, according to research from Ohio University.[23] The average person will burn about 150 extra calories following a metabolic strength workout.

You tone where it counts.

The Turn Up Your Fat Burn metabolic circuit hits every major muscle group. You're shaping some of your body's biggest trouble zones, including your arms, shoulders, chest, abs, hips, butt, and thighs. As the weeks progress, you'll start to work several of these muscles simultaneously for a bigger metabolic boost. Working your arms and legs together, for example, puts more stress on your body, which in turn produces higher levels of muscle-building hormones like

IGF-1, growth hormone, and testosterone, all of which influence metabolic rate while stimulating both protein synthesis and fat burning.

If you're a woman who is concerned about adding bulk, don't be: Women really don't have the ability to add a lot of muscle mass, and it would take very heavy weights anyway. These circuits use primarily lighter weights so both men and women are mostly improving muscle tone.

You continue to surprise your muscles.

Each week you'll do a different circuit, shocking your muscles in a new and good way. This progression, a type of training known as undulating or nonlinear periodization, keeps your muscles surprised so they respond better. Research has shown that this type of workout program is significantly more effective at boosting strength than workouts that vary the routine only every month or so.[24] Variety is also a lot more interesting: Your mind and your muscles won't get as bored when you mix things up more often.

You save time.

When you do a typical strength workout, you perform a move for 30 seconds, followed by a long recovery time—often up to 90 seconds. In an hour-long workout, you might work only 20 minutes. With a metabolic strength circuit, you're flipping that equation and working for much longer than you're recovering. You may still be doing 20 minutes of work, but now you'll be finished in 30 to 45 minutes.

BOOSTING YOUR VT1

In the last chapter, we took a look at Ventilatory Threshold 1 and how this marker can be used to improve the amount of fat you're burning through your workout. You'll get a chance to determine your unique VT1 in Chapter 5. But first, let's answer the question: What does it take to raise your VT1 level?

Panel Approved:
"It worked for us!"

Here's what some of our test panelists had to say about the metabolic strength circuits.

"This was a completely different way of strength training for me. I usually just went to the gym and sat around between exercises. Moving from one exercise to the next felt so much better. Before I never put my full effort into doing that second or third set; here it was like a fresh start with each cycle!"

—LISA MILLER

"I never really did much strength training before, and whatever I did do was usually on the machines at the gym, which never felt like much of a challenge. But these circuits definitely gave me a good workout! My heart rate was up the whole time, and I was working up a sweat."

—SUSAN MAUSER

"My mother had osteoporosis, so I know it's important to do strength training for my bones, but I never really got that into it. I liked the challenge of these circuits: I started out with some 5-pound weights, but before too long, I got a set of 7s and 10s—it was great being able to make more progress with each week!"

—WENDY KLEMKA

"I loved that each week the circuit was a little different from the one before. It wasn't just a matter of doing the same old exercises with more weight or reps. You're really working all of your muscles in different ways, and you're done in less than 45 minutes!"

—LESLIE KINGSTON

"I really liked mixing up the different strength moves. It wasn't just going out and lifting a weight for as many times as you can; it was lifting that weight while trying to balance on one leg. The flow of the strength exercises made the whole workout much more interesting."

—PETE BROWN

The best way to improve your aerobic fitness and bump your VT1 is through a unique type of interval training. Intervals are hot right now. You'll see them in group exercise classes at the gym, in fitness and health magazines, and as part of most trainers' prescriptions for their clients. They're popular for a reason: They work.

With most interval training plans, you work at a period of increased effort or intensity for a relatively short time (anywhere from a few seconds to a few minutes), followed immediately by a recovery period that allows you to catch your breath before doing another work interval. Some interval plans are designed around bursts of very high effort levels followed by longer recovery periods. These plans, often known as high-intensity interval training (HIIT), or anaerobic intervals, are designed to push the lactate threshold—the VT2 level at which your body accumulates lactic acid and its by-products. They're fantastic if you're training for an athletic event like a road race or triathlon, or if you take part in sports that require bursts of intensity followed by recovery, like tennis, hockey, basketball, or soccer.

But if your goal is to lose body fat, high-intensity intervals won't help you become a more efficient fat burner. Instead, you need to do aerobic intervals—exercise that burns both fat and carbs—so your body learns to burn that fat more efficiently.

By doing work intervals that push you slightly beyond your VT1, which is your fat-burning sweet spot, you'll ultimately push your VT1 level higher. Researchers in France found that among out-of-shape older adults, VT1 levels improved by 26 percent after a 3-month interval-training program using walk/jog sessions on a track twice a week. Maximal oxygen uptake (a measure of fitness) also improved by 20 percent.[25]

Intervals create an overload to which the body needs to adapt. By pushing with small doses of slightly higher intensity for short-to-moderate durations, then pulling back before you get too tired, you'll still be working at an aerobic (i.e., fat-burning) level but with enough intensity to produce a real training effect. So even though you might not be burning as many calories as with a high-intensity interval, you're teaching your body to tolerate more stress while still efficiently using fat as its main fuel source. As you progress, you'll keep those fat-burning levels high and won't switch over to carbs as the primary fuel source.

The benefits continue when you're not exercising. Even if you exercise for 3 hours a week, there are another 165 hours a week when your body remains mostly at rest. As we briefly mentioned in the last chapter, by shifting your VT1 level higher and training your body with regular exercise, you'll burn not only more calories from fat during the workout but more fat all day long through an elevated resting metabolism. Assuming you're following a sensible diet, you'll be burning more fat during the day—about 4 percent more after just 4 weeks, according to research.[26]

In addition to boosting your fitness levels, intervals will burn calories more efficiently than a steady-pace workout like a power walk. A 30-minute walk/jog interval will burn between 25 and 43 percent more calories than just walking briskly for the same length of time.

Work and Rest Ratios

A key to interval training is to progressively increase how long you're working at a higher intensity and reducing how long you have to recover. These work-to-recovery ratios can shift as you become better trained. With the Turn Up Your Fat Burn interval workouts, you'll move between zone 1 (recovery) and zone 2 (work interval).

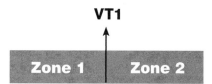

Example:

WORK-TO-REST INTERVAL RATIO	WORK (ZONE 2)	RECOVERY (ZONE 1)
1:2	4 minutes > VT1	8 minutes < VT1
1:1	4 minutes > VT1	4 minutes < VT1
2:1	4 minutes > VT1	2 minutes < VT1
3:1	4 minutes > VT1	1 minute 20 seconds < VT1
4:1	4 minutes > VT1	1 minute < VT1

With the Turn Up Your Fat Burn program, you do two or three cardio workouts a week, almost all of them including fat-burning intervals that consistently push you to work just beyond VT1 before giving you some time to recover before working harder again. In the first week, you'll work for 3 minutes during each interval, then recover for 4 minutes at a lower intensity, a work-to-recovery ratio of 3:4. For Week 2, the intervals become as long as the rest time—4 minutes each (a 4:4, also known as a 1:1, ratio). And in Week 3, the intervals become slightly longer than the recovery—5 minutes of work with a 4-minute rest interval (5:4 ratio). As your fitness progresses, you'll find it easier to maintain this higher intensity longer.

In the final week of the program, you'll move beyond VT1 with some brief (20-second) bursts at a much higher intensity (anaerobic intervals) that get you closer to VT2 (also known as your lactate threshold). Incorporating these short speed bursts will give you just a bit more of a butt-kicking in the final week. It also will help move you closer to your VT2, which will also ultimately improve your overall fitness.

YOUR ULTIMATE FAT-BLASTING EQUATION

Turn Up Your Fat Burn's combination of metabolic strength circuits to build lean muscle and VT1 interval training to boost your fat-burning level is designed to maximize how much body fat you're torching each

Panel Approved:
"It worked for us!"

Here's what some of our test panelists had to say about the interval workouts.

"I felt like I had so much more energy by doing the intervals. And having a set goal, like increasing my intensity for just a few minutes at a time, made the workouts go by much faster."

—ANNE JENKINS

"Before I started following the Turn Up Your Fat Burn program, I would run 3 miles in about 35 minutes at a steady pace. By picking up my speed during the intervals, I was able to run farther in less time. It gave me the most bang for my buck, which—as a working mother of three—is what I've been looking for. I don't have a lot of time to devote to my workouts, so getting a good calorie-burning session in a minimum amount of time is key!"

—CINDY WENRICH

"I loved the challenge of intervals, being able to get my intensity up for just a relatively short time and then having a chance to recover. And progressing each week made me feel like I was getting more fit with each workout!"

—LISA MILLER

"Intervals are great for motivation because you know you have to do them only for a short while. The idea of going out for a 35-minute run seems hard mentally, but when you break it into these intervals, it's much more doable."

—KIMBERLY HAMPSEY

"I've found that after doing a few interval workouts, my heart rate recovers much more quickly. It's getting easier, which I guess means my conditioning is getting better!"

—CATHERINE SCHAPER

and every day, both in the workouts themselves and long afterward. Each week you'll be able to burn more and more fat as the workouts progress, and you'll fine-tune your fitness levels to maximize metabolism and fat burn.

Over the next 4 weeks, your metabolic strength circuits and cardio VT1 interval routines will get progressively more challenging. In the Week 1 metabolic strength circuit, the focus is on basic strength moves like deadlifts, squats, lunges, and chest presses. For the cardio, you have a slightly longer recovery time than a work interval. With Week 2, the strength exercises become a little more challenging; now you'll start to combine different moves, like adding a shoulder press to your deadlift or a triceps press to your squat. Working more muscles simultaneously will kick up your heart rate while maximizing your results. In the interval workout, work and recovery times are mostly equal.

In Week 3, you'll add in some jumping (plyometric) exercises to your metabolic strength workout to boost your heart rate, along with some balancing exercises to improve your sense of balance while also strengthening your core muscles. During the cardio, you'll have slightly less recovery time, compared with the work interval. And in Week 4, you'll add compound sets to your strength routine, working two exercises per muscle group with different types of movements. This final circuit routine will "shock" and strengthen your muscles in a whole new way, but after the previous weeks, you'll be ready for it. Meanwhile, we'll take the cardio intervals up another notch, this time getting close to VT2 for very short bursts of speed followed by recovery near VT1, which will challenge your aerobic fitness and help you achieve the results you want.

Fat-Fighting Facts

○ You don't have to grunt and groan with heavy dumbbells to see results. A recent study from McMaster University found that lifting light weights (about 30 percent of maximum effort, or about 24 times until fatigue) was just as effective at building muscles as heavier ones (up to 90 percent maximum load, or about 5 to 10 reps before fatigue), as long as the person was able to fully fatigue the target muscle group by the final rep.[27]

○ The more active you are, the more likely you are to push yourself during a workout. Researchers from New Zealand found that women who exercised regularly were more likely on their own to work at a heart rate near and above VT1 than their more sedentary counterparts.[28]

○ When it comes to the amount of fat you'll burn during a workout, you'll torch more of it going for a run than you would hopping on a bike, according to a British study from the University of Birmingham.[29]

○ Slow and steady doesn't always win the race for weight loss. New research from the University of Florida shows that women who lost about 1½ pounds a week or more were more successful at achieving long-term significant weight loss than those who lost ½ pound a week or less. The fast-weight losers were five times more likely to have lost at least 10 percent of their body weight at 18 months than those who took off the pounds more gradually.[30]

○ Exercise is key to keeping off dangerous belly fat. Subjects in a study from the University of Alabama at Birmingham who had lost an average of 24 pounds and kept up their fitness routine of either strength or cardio for 40 minutes twice a week, for 1 year, gained absolutely no visceral fat, even if they gained a little weight back. Those who had stopped exercise altogether weren't so lucky: They averaged about a 33 percent increase in visceral fat.[31]

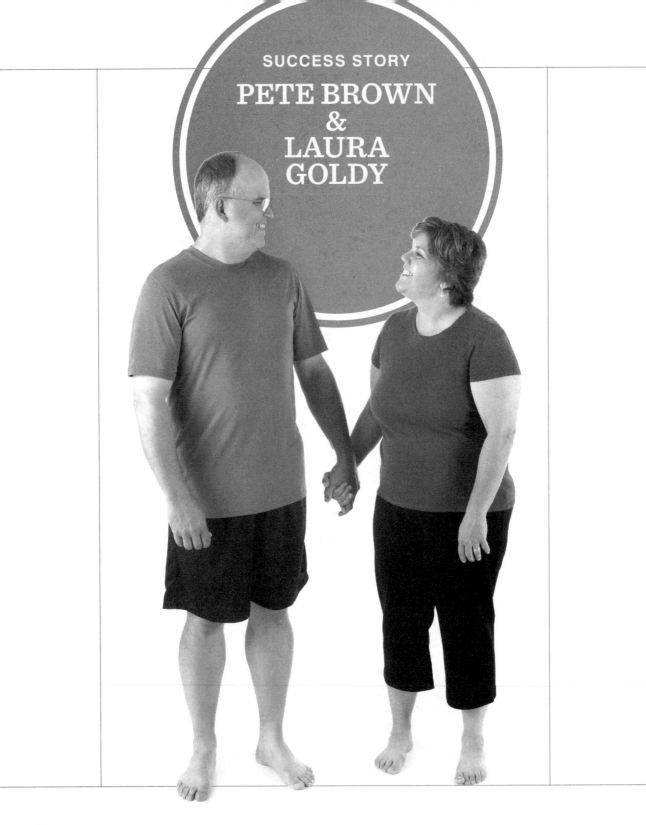

SUCCESS STORY
PETE BROWN
&
LAURA
GOLDY

PETE

Age: 48

Height: 5'9"

Pounds lost: $21^1/_2$

Inches lost: $3^1/_2$

What he's most proud of: "I'm wearing clothes I haven't been able to fit into in years!"

Favorite foods: Ham and turkey in a whole wheat wrap; almond snack packs

LAURA

Age: 49

Height: 5'0"

Pounds lost: 6

Inches lost: 2

What she's most proud of: "The changes I see in myself—not just physical ones but also making better lifestyle choices."

Favorite foods: Wheat Thins with hummus or avocado spread; Fiber One cereal bars

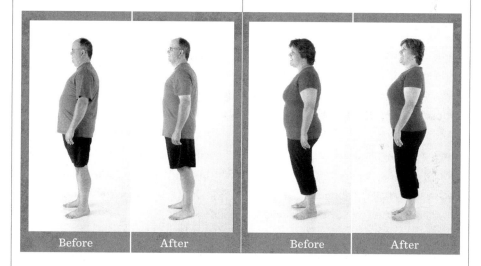

Before   After   Before   After

Pete Brown and Laura Goldy have shared many things over their 22 years together—raising three healthy children, building a happy home, celebrating successful careers in finance and education. They've also shared a weight problem.

"We started doing Weight Watchers together before we got married, and at the time I lost about 40 pounds and Laura lost another 20," says Pete. But over the years, in a life where family activities were often celebrated and centered around food, both began to put the

continued

PETE & LAURA *continued*

weight back on. "We both grew up with large families that celebrated events with traditional, big meals. When we get together, it's a big food and drink fest!" says Laura.

But recently, both Laura and Pete realized there needed to be change. "I was looking through some pictures and realized I didn't like what I had become," says Laura, whose starting weight on the plan was almost 187 pounds. "I'll be 50 next year, and I want to feel good about myself."

Pete had a similar "aha" moment: "I looked in the mirror and knew that I didn't want to be that guy who couldn't even see his neck anymore," says Pete, whose starting weight was 247 pounds. "And I was worried about my health—I have a family history of heart disease and diabetes, and I didn't want to increase my risk any further."

Although they mostly did their workouts separately, the two compared notes about the strength moves and interval segments. Pete hit the elliptical machine in the basement in the morning to do his cardio, and Laura did her intervals outside, walking and jogging on a quarter-mile loop. While Pete had done some strength workouts before, he'd never incorporated balancing exercises or combo moves like the ones in the cir-

cuit routines. "It was a totally different kind of workout, and it was really motivating to challenge myself with all these new moves."

"I could tell my endurance was greatly improved," adds Laura. "I used to be gasping for air when I jogged in the park, and now I can breathe a lot easier. And I liked being able to measure my intensity using just my breathing as a guide."

The couple also supported each other at the dining room table. "We both have really busy schedules, so we tried to pick foods that were healthy but convenient," says Laura. That meant lots of salads, lean protein like salmon or chicken, and simple snacks like whole grain crackers with hummus. "I've always been a meat-and-potatoes kind of guy, but I found myself really enjoying a lot of vegetarian meals," adds Pete.

After a month on the program, Pete had dropped more than 21 pounds and lost an inch off his waist. "I had to dig in my closet to find a belt that fit, because the ones I was using didn't have holes that were small enough!" says Pete. And his resting heart rate, which was surprisingly high at the start of his program, dropped by nearly 20 percent.

For Laura, the weight loss has been

more gradual, but she's still reaping the payoffs. "My pants are all much looser around the waist and butt," she says, "although I'm still working toward one favorite pair of jeans that I can't wait to wear again!" And after a month on the plan, her new profile photo on Facebook drew approving comments from friends: "One asked whether I'd edited my picture, because I looked so good!" Pete added, "We went to visit our son at college who had not seen either of us since we started the program, and he was so pleased and surprised at our results!"

Both found the benefits of the workouts spilled into other areas of their lives. "My job can get pretty stressful, and I realized I was much more relaxed after I exercised," says Pete. He also found his acid reflux symptoms were greatly reduced, and he hopes to reduce and even get off his medication altogether. Laura found that she was much more alert and energetic after her workouts.

But perhaps most important, Pete and Laura say they want to be good role models for their 10-year-old daughter, Kelly, who has her own weight concerns.

"It's our job to teach her some healthy habits that will last," says Pete. "She's definitely noticed the changes in our eating habits and is making a conscious effort to eat more healthy foods and be more active." Kelly's even begun riding her bike while Laura does her walk/runs in the park.

Four months after the last "official" weigh-in, Pete reports being down a total of 35 pounds and continues to exercise faithfully most mornings before work. "I feel good about how I look for the first time in a long time," he says. "I've gotten a lot of compliments." One of the biggest lifestyle changes he's stuck with has been to cut alcohol consumption down to no more than three drinks a week. "I used to eat a lot at parties or dinners out after I had a couple of cocktails, and I think cutting back has helped me stay on track."

Laura has dropped about 10 pounds and is proudly fitting into pants that are one full size smaller than those she wore before starting the program. "This has been the starting block to getting us into a healthier mode," adds Laura. "We've made some changes in our home, and we want to continue them."

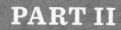

PART II

Before You Begin

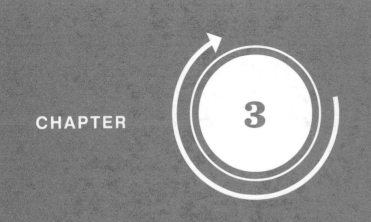

CHAPTER 3

Preparing for Maximum Fat Burn

We've provided a lot of information to digest about why the Turn Up Your Fat Burn program works and what sets it apart from every other fitness program you've read about or tried. You're almost ready to lace up your sneakers and grab your weights, hit the treadmill, or head outside to begin. But first you need to get a handle on the basics of a successful workout.

WORKOUT PLANNING

When will you work out? How can you fit this into your schedule? What will you do if you feel sore afterward? It really helps to have a plan!

Scheduling strategies

When should you work out? The easy answer: whenever it works best for you. These workouts are designed to be brief; most take no more than 35 to 45 minutes. If you have more time on one day and want to combine a cardio and strength program into one longer workout, go for it. If you want to split it up and do one in the morning and one later in the day, that's fine, too. (Many experts recommend mornings over evenings, if only to avoid some of the roadblocks and distractions that can circumvent your workout plans as the day progresses.)

If you'd rather stagger workouts throughout the week, that's also great. Actually, that's better. Since each workout will boost your metabolism for a few hours postexercise, you'll get a more significant afterburn by spacing them out. The object, though, is to fit these workouts into your schedule. The only hard-and-fast rule: Do not do the strength workout 2 days in a row. Your muscles need time to recover and grow, so give yourself at least 36 to 48 hours between metabolic strength workouts.

Combining cardio and strength workouts

It's totally fine if you need to save some time one week by combining your workouts. As to which should come first—cardio or strength—the research varies. Some studies show that starting with resistance training boosts the way the body burns fat and increases overall calorie burn, but you could compromise your workout by raising your heart rate past your VT1 heart rate before you even begin. Then again, performing cardio first can fatigue some muscles before strength training starts.

In order to keep your VT1 level as accurate as possible, we suggest doing the cardio first. If you're breaking it up and doing one workout in the morning and the other later in the day, the order won't matter.

Easing soreness

Some muscle soreness is actually positive—it shows you've been challenging yourself. Resistance training creates tiny tears in the muscles fibers. When your body repairs those microtears, the muscles grow stronger. However, they can make you feel a bit achy when you sit a while, go down stairs, or just move around.

If you're experiencing mild muscle soreness, try applying ice to the affected area. Keep it on no longer than 10 to 15 minutes at a time. You might even consider hopping into a tub filled with cold water. There's some evidence that cold water causes blood vessels to constrict, decreasing inflammation. Try to avoid taking a very hot shower or bath immediately after your workout, as this can increase inflammation. You may also find it helpful to spend a few extra minutes cooling down and stretching after exercising.

Also try gently massaging your muscles, using a little lotion or massage oil. For a sore spot on a small area like your neck or shoulder, simply apply gentle pressure using a thumb or finger. Knead larger muscles with your hands. A foam roller can also be helpful. This long, dense tube, which resembles a superthick pool noodle, can help break up deep scar tissue and is relatively inexpensive ($15 to $30). The roller is especially good for tight areas like the hips, butt, shoulders, and back.

Nonprescription medications like ibuprofen (Motrin or Advil), naproxen (Aleve), and acetaminophen (Tylenol) can reduce inflammation in muscles, joints, and connective tissue. But be careful—taking too many of these meds can lead to stomach, liver, or kidney problems. Talk to your doctor if you find yourself taking this medicine more than once or twice a week.

There's also evidence of relief beyond the bottle. A study reported in the *Journal of Pain* found that consuming 2 grams of ginger a day reduced pain caused by exercise by 25 percent.[1] Other research has shown that omega-3 fatty acids (found in cold-water fish, walnuts, and flaxseed, among other sources) are a natural anti-inflammatory, as is quercetin, a phytochemical found in apples and red onion, among other foods.

Also be sure to drink plenty of water, which will help flush waste products associated with muscle soreness out of your body. To determine how much water you should be sipping, weigh yourself before exercising (go to the bathroom first) and then afterward (again, if you have to pee, do it before you hop on the scale). Then rehydrate at 125 to 150 percent of the volume change. In other words, if you weigh ½ pound less after exercising, that's about 8 ounces, so drink 10 to 12 ounces of water postworkout.

STRENGTH BASICS

If you haven't done strength training in a while, you can expect to feel a little muscle soreness 12 to 48 hours after you work out. Think of it as a "good" pain—it lets you know that you've challenged yourself and are getting ready to build more lean muscle. (See the previous section for more on muscle soreness.)

If you're having trouble with any of the strength exercises, feel free to modify them. If you find any of these moves too difficult, use a lighter weight or go back to an earlier week's exercise; for example, do a regular squat or deadlift instead of a single leg one. If you feel uncertain about progressing to the next week, remain at the current week or try to complete an additional day of the same week's workout. Also, for some exercises, we've added suggestions on how to make the move easier.

Watch your form

It's more important to get your technique right than to bang out all the reps of an exercise—we want you healthier at the end of the 4 weeks than when you started!

Form—the correct movement for each exercise—is very important during strength training. Poor form isn't just ineffective; it can lead to injury.

It's a good idea to train in a room that has a mirror so you can see exactly what you are doing. Notes panelist Leslie Kingston, "I found it very important to have a mirror handy while I was exercising. I often found myself looking at my form and then making some much-needed tweaks. It gave me instant feedback and made a big difference in the quality of my workout!"

Follow a few rules of thumb when doing the strength moves.

Shoulders down: Bring your shoulders all the way up to your ears. Feel funny? Now press them all the way down. That's the position they should be in whenever you're lifting weights. It's also a good rule to follow when you're not lifting weights, so you don't end up with back or neck pain.

Stay centered: Don't lean too far forward, especially during squats and lunges. For most lunges and squats, keep your weight over your heels. If you look down, you should see your toes, not your knees. Bringing your knees past your toes puts too much pressure on the joint.

Wear a girdle: An imaginary one, of course. Your transverse abdominals are the deepest abdominal muscle group, and they wrap around your trunk like a corset. Think about keeping these muscles engaged, especially during standing exercises and prone moves like planks. To activate these muscles, pull your belly button in, as if you were trying to slip on a pair of too-tight jeans.

Don't lock it out: Avoid locking your elbows or knees during the exercises to prevent injury to the joints.

Just breathe

Try not to hold your breath at any point during an exercise. In general, exhale on the exertion (lifting the weight) and inhale while you recover. When you hold your breath, you will not only be uncomfortable but may get dizzy. By breathing evenly through any movement, you'll feel more relaxed and responsive, which makes the exercise feel easier.

Find the right tempo

Control your speed of movement when performing repetitions. Go too fast and momentum—not your muscles—does most of the work. Go too slow and the movement can become more difficult (and you can actually feel sorer the next day). A full repetition (lifting and lowering the weight one time) should take about four counts—two to lift and two to lower.

Pick the best weight

Use a weight heavy enough that you feel it in the belly of the muscle you're trying to work (not the joints), but not so heavy that you can barely get through the exercise without shaking or feeling completely worn out. The right weight is highly individual: For many beginners, the starting weight may range from 5 to 10 pounds, depending on the exercise. You should be able to perform "quality" repetitions—no swaying, jerking, or swinging—for the entire length of each exercise. Don't force the movement by leaning back or using momentum.

FLEXIBILITY BASICS

Stretching is an important but often ignored part of a workout. Although recent research has sparked some controversy regarding the benefits of stretching before a workout, many fitness experts swear by it. Here's what you should know.

Static stretching

Most of us think of stretching as leaning over and holding a muscle for 20 to 30 seconds. That's called static stretching. Several studies have shown that static stretching before exercise doesn't help much. In fact, a recent study of more than 1,400 runners, conducted by USA Track and Field, found that those who stretched before their runs over a 3-month period had exactly the same injury rate (about 16 percent) as those who didn't take the time to stretch.[2]

So why bother with static stretching? For one, stretching clearly improves range of motion, and the more ease of movement you have, the easier it is to do everyday activities, whether you're reaching up for a can on the top shelf, changing a lightbulb, or bending down to pick up stray socks. Also, the more range of motion you have, the more easily you may be able to do activities like running, swimming, and cycling.

Research has also shown that static stretching after a workout may help reduce muscle soreness. One recent study found that subjects who practiced static stretching after a strength workout had significantly greater range of motion and faster recovery of muscle strength than those who did not stretch at all.[3]

Finally, if your muscles are very tight, static stretches may decrease your risk of injury. That's especially true of the hamstrings and hips, where too-tight muscles can lead to back pain.

Dynamic stretching

The other major type of stretching, one that's become more popular in the fitness world, is dynamic stretching. You move a muscle through its full range of motion several times—there's no "stretch and hold." Arm circles, leg raises, knee lifts, and heel kicks fall into the dynamic school of stretching.

Athletes often use dynamic stretches before an event or practice to mimic the motions of their sport. There's some evidence that dynamic stretching before a weight workout can help increase power. A Japanese study found that people who did a series of dynamic stretching before a weight routine had about a 12 percent increase in power; when they did static stretching before a workout, they showed no increase in muscle power.[4] Other studies have also shown improvements in agility and high-speed running performance after a dynamic warmup.[5]

Building stretching into your workout

Ideally, do a brief warmup, and then spend a few minutes doing some dynamic stretching before your strength or cardio routine. When you're finished, take a couple of minutes more to do some static stretching to help improve your flexibility.

Always warm up for a few minutes with some light jogging or even just marching in place. Warming up the muscles increases bloodflow and raises the temperature in the muscles, which will make them more elastic and pliable.

When doing static stretches, don't go past the point of slight discomfort. You want to feel the stretch but not pain. For dynamic stretches, don't bounce into the movement—keep it controlled and steady.

CARDIO BASICS

Cardiovascular (aka aerobic or cardio) exercise is crucial for weight loss, fitness, and better health. The good news is that you don't have to run marathons, gasp for air, or train for hours a week to get results. Just 30 minutes a day of consistent cardiovascular training (enough to keep you at least slightly breathless) can have significant results. In fact, the U.S. Department of Health and Human Services says adults need a minimum of $2\frac{1}{2}$ hours of moderate exercise (or 75 minutes of vigorous activity) a week to achieve good health.[6]

Does the type of cardio matter?

Not really, although for the first couple of weeks, it helps to do the same type of exercise as your VT1 test (coming up in Chapter 5), so you know how fast or hard to exercise during the "work" part of the interval. If you reach VT1 during your test at 4.0 mph and a 3 percent incline on the treadmill, you'll know to speed it up a little more (say, 4.2 mph) or boost the incline to 4 percent during the interval.

Once you get used to what it feels like to push just past VT1 (your speech is choppy and you need to breathe frequently, but you're not gasping for air), you can take your workout to a different machine or type of exercise.

How hard should I work?

When you're excited about a new workout, it's tempting to go all out and give it your max. While we're thrilled that you've decided to join us on this journey, we don't want you to burn out or get injured.

Research shows that more than half of exercisers give up because they believe their program is too difficult. On the other hand, if you take things too easy, you won't see much in the way of positive results.

You want to exercise at a level high enough that you can improve your fitness and health but not so high that you quit in frustration. This is another reason to love intervals—they allow you to challenge yourself for brief periods without burning out. Remember, with the Turn Up

Your Fat Burn workouts, we focus on fat-burning exercise, which means you'll rarely go into the anaerobic (ultra-high-intensity) level of training. For the cardio workouts, you'll work on three different levels. Warmup and cooldown should be fairly easy, enough to break a light sweat. For the intervals, you'll alternate between a somewhat hard level and a moderate level.

How can you tell if you're working at the right level? There are a few methods, but let's focus for now on rate of perceived exertion, or RPE. If you've been to the gym in the last few years or picked up a fitness magazine, you've probably heard of RPE. You simply rank your exercise intensity based on your perception of your overall effort, including how hard it is to breathe, how tired your muscles feel, and your mental status. The beauty of RPE is that it's applicable to any activity—running, walking, swimming, cycling, skating, or using the elliptical trainer or stairclimber. It isn't tied to a set speed, resistance, or incline.

Exercise physiologists rank perceived exertion on a scale of 6 to 20, but to keep it simple, we use a scale of 1 to 10. At 1, you're sitting back on the couch with your feet up on the coffee table. At 10, you're sprinting for your life away from a knife-wielding serial killer (or maybe just sprinting for a bus that's about to pull away from the stop). It's difficult for most of us to stay at 10 for more than a few seconds.

During the Turn Up Your Fat Burn cardio workouts, you'll want to

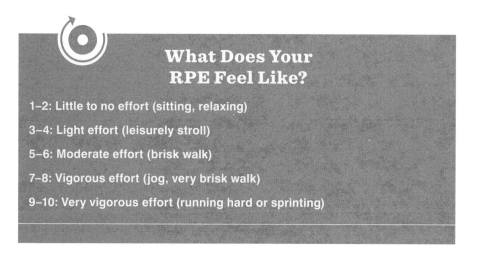

What Does Your RPE Feel Like?

1–2: Little to no effort (sitting, relaxing)

3–4: Light effort (leisurely stroll)

5–6: Moderate effort (brisk walk)

7–8: Vigorous effort (jog, very brisk walk)

9–10: Very vigorous effort (running hard or sprinting)

keep your warmup at an RPE of 3 or 4. You're doing some work, but it's fairly easy. When you get into the intervals, aim for 7 or 8 on the higher end—hard, but not so hard that you couldn't keep it up for at least a few minutes. When you recover, you'll want to be at about 5. You can catch your breath, but you're still definitely putting forth a good effort.

If you're still unsure whether you're working at the right intensity, we'll discuss some other monitoring methods in Chapter 5, when we get into the cardio workout details in more depth.

GET THE GEAR

We've designed the Turn Up Your Fat Burn program to be done anywhere, anytime, at your convenience, but you will need some basic equipment to get started.

Weights: If you're exercising at home, at a minimum you'll need one set of light-to-medium dumbbells and one set of medium-to-heavy dumbbells. For most of us, that means a range of 5 to 15 pounds, depending on fitness level and ability. Try to use a weight that will challenge you by the final rep while you're still maintaining good form (no hip swaying, back bending, or overall jerking allowed!).

Timing device (optional): You can always look at the clock on the wall, but using a watch with a timer or second hand is a better way to track just how long you are resting between strength exercises or doing your cardio program. Timing is important during the 4-week plan, when you need to time your exertion/recovery cycles.

Heart rate monitor (optional): We also strongly recommend using a heart rate monitor. If you have one already, great! If not, consider purchasing one (a basic model will cost less than $50). This device isn't absolutely necessary, but it can help you more precisely determine your appropriate training levels.

Weight bench, sturdy chair, or mat: While not a necessity, a weight bench can be helpful for several exercises that require you to either lie down or step up on a sturdy platform. You can also use a step bench, the kind used in step aerobics classes. If you don't have either a bench or

No Weights at Home?

No worries! A lot of ordinary things around the house can take the place of dumbbells. Here's a sampling of what you might find and their approximate weights.

½-liter water bottle or soup can filled, 1 pound

1-liter water bottle filled, 2 pounds

½-gallon milk jug filled, 4 pounds

1-gallon milk jug filled, 8 pounds

step, a sturdy chair can fill in for seated and kneeling moves, and you can use a sofa cushion or other large pillow for the exercises done lying down. Finally, a yoga mat or other nonslippery floor mat can provide helpful cushioning during floor exercises.

Workout shoes: Haven't bought new sneakers in a while? Now's the time. The right athletic shoes will support your feet, keep you comfortable, and reduce your risk of injury by providing enough cushioning and stability. Pick a pair designed for your favorite activity. If you plan to walk, get walking shoes; if you're more of a runner, invest in running shoes. If you plan to do both, opt for running shoes—they'll do a better job of protecting your joints against the impact of running.

You can wear either running or walking shoes for the strength exercises, but avoid supersimple slip-ons like Keds. They're cute, but they don't provide enough support for your muscles and joints. You don't have to shell out the big bucks to get a good pair of shoes. Most sporting-goods chains and online retailers like Amazon or Zappos sell supportive (and stylish!) athletic shoes for less than $50. You may want to get fitted at a running or sporting goods store where knowledgeable sales clerks can help you pick the best features for the types of workouts you like to do.

Apparel: Next up for the ladies: a good-fitting sports bra. Trust us, it's worth every penny. The right support up front can make all the difference between feeling strong and wishing you were finished *this minute.* If you're on the larger size, consider getting a bra that has separate cups rather than the old compression variety. You'll not only avoid uniboob, you'll also feel (and look) a whole lot better, especially if you're doing a high-impact activity like jogging.

Finally, get a T-shirt or two and some shorts or tights made of a wicking fabric, which is engineered to move moisture away from your skin. Dry-F.I.T., Coolmax, polypropylene, and even certain types of wool are engineered to keep you dry and comfy. Cotton may be great when you're kicking back on the couch or hitting the hay, but when you're working out, it can be a killer. Cotton absorbs perspiration and can turn even your lightest T-shirt into a clammy mess after you start to sweat. In the summer, it will weigh you down; in the winter, it can make you chilled.

FOOD BASICS

It will come as no surprise to anyone who has ever stepped on a scale that to lose weight, the number of calories taken in must be less than the number of calories burned off. Our 4-week plan burns about 1,000 calories a week, depending on your size and the intensity of your exercising. You will burn a significant percentage of those calories from fat tissue. But in order to see results in your waistline as well as your fitness level, you need to make the right food choices as part of the plan.

In Part IV, we'll give you plenty of details about what you should eat to boost your metabolism and keep your fat-burning engines revved up. The good news is that we won't ask you to cut out entire food groups, send you on some wacky cayenne pepper juice fast, or force you to follow annoying rules like not eating after the sun goes down or never enjoying a piece of bread again. Here's what you will find: a healthy, well-balanced nutrition program that includes plenty of your favorite foods (including fast food options!), plus snacks and desserts. For the best results, be sure to review those chapters before you begin the 4-week plan.

Even if you don't follow the meal plan to the letter, take a little time to become more aware of what fuel you're putting in your body. For starters, there's no time like the present to purge some of the junk from your house. Consider which temptations often lead you astray and clear them out. Don't just hide the ice cream in the back of the freezer or the cookies on the bottom shelf of your pantry. Get the stuff out of the house—give it to a friend with kids, offer it to a neighbor, or send it to your kid's school as a snack. Know your trigger foods, and get rid of them. This way you won't be tempted by readily available high-calorie treats once you start the 4-week plan.

Now is also a good time to stock up on healthy foods. Don't worry, you don't have to spend a fortune. Picking up a few basics will make it a lot easier to prepare healthy meals for your entire family. Load up on whole grains like whole wheat bread and pasta, brown rice, and oats. Peruse the produce aisle for a variety of vegetables and fruits, including some you may not have tried in a while, if ever. Don't forget the dairy aisle. Low-fat or fat-free yogurt and cheese are key sources of calcium in your diet and also provide plenty of protein without a ton of fat or calories.

You might also experiment with some new foods like agave nectar, a natural sweetener considered sweeter than sugar and not as processed, as well as products like flaxseed crackers and soy cheese, which are suggested (though not mandatory) on the meal plan.

The workouts in the Turn Up Your Fat Burn program are designed to help you burn more fat all day long and boost your metabolism, but exercise isn't the only way to rev your calorie-burning engines. Certain foods and eating behaviors can also help raise your metabolism and ability to burn fat efficiently. You can start today by following these three basic nutrition rules.

Rule #1: Drink 8 to 10 glasses of cold water daily.

You've probably heard about the 8-glasses-a-day idea. It's based on a recommendation from the Institute of Medicine (an independent group that advises the government) that women consume 11$\frac{1}{2}$ cups of fluid a day and men consume 15$\frac{1}{2}$ cups.[7] At least 20 percent of the total typically comes from food, which takes the amount to drink down to about 9 cups. A cup isn't much—just 8 ounces, less than a typical can of soda.

If the fluid is cold, your metabolism actually perks up a bit. A study published in the *Journal of Clinical Endocrinology and Metabolism* found that the participants burned an additional 50 calories per day by drinking 1.5 liters of cold water.[8] Choosing cold fluid is important because your body warms it during digestion, accounting for 60 to 70 percent of the energy burn.

If you can't stomach the thought of drinking 8 to 9 glasses of plain water, you can include flavored seltzer (check labels; the only ingredients should be natural flavor and carbonated water). Or flavor water yourself with slices of lemon, lime, or cucumber. Just be sure to keep the calorie count low while avoiding artificial sweeteners.

Rule #2: Eat breakfast.

Starting off the day with breakfast can help you manage your weight and eat less throughout the day. Take your cue from the National Weight Control Registry, which follows folks who have lost at least 30 pounds and kept it off for a year (or more!). Of these people, 78 percent eat breakfast every day.[9] Other long-term studies report that those who skip breakfast are heavier than those who make time for a morning nosh. The logic: When you skip breakfast, you're far more likely to overcompensate with extra calories later in the day. You also slow down your metabolism instead of giving it a jump start in the morning.

Our 4-week plan includes a filling breakfast with plenty of fiber. Until you start the program, just be sure to begin your day with something nourishing, even if it's just a small bowl of cereal with milk or a banana and a small yogurt.

Rule #3: Eat at regular intervals.

Eat more and still lose weight? Sounds too good to be true. When you skip breakfast, skimp on lunch, and then are starving by dinnertime, you're likely to consume way more calories in an evening's binge than you would have eaten in a few small, healthy meals throughout the day.

Try not to go more than 4 or 5 hours between meals. Small snacks will help you get more out of your workouts and boost your metabolism, so you'll burn more calories every day. A study from Georgia State University presented at the 2005 annual meeting of the American College of Sports Medicine found that when athletes ate snacks of 250 calories each, three times a day, they performed better than when they went snack free. Researchers also found that when subjects snacked, they ate less at each of their three regular meals, so their overall calorie intake for the day was actually lower.[10]

When you skip meals, your metabolism slows down, so when you're ready to dive facefirst into a plate of pasta, your body wants to hold each and every calorie near and dear. Over time, this can contribute to weight gain (and make you very grumpy).

BURT DUREN

Age: 51

Height: 6'0"

Pounds lost: $22\frac{1}{2}$

Inches lost: $6\frac{3}{4}$

What he's most proud of: "I've busted out of my exercise rut and finally lost some stubborn pounds. I'm also able to reduce my diabetes medications."

Favorite Foods: Fat-free microwave popcorn; almonds; low-fat yogurt

By most people's standards, Burt Duren was in pretty good shape when he joined the Turn Up Your Fat Burn panel. He rode a stationary bike in his basement for 40 minutes 3 mornings a week and lifted weights a couple of times a week. But he wasn't losing much weight—in fact, with each passing year, he'd put on a few more pounds. Soon the number on the scale was dangerously close to 250. "I was active, but it wasn't the right kind of active," he says. "I needed to kick things up a notch."

As a vice president in finance, Burt's no stranger to numbers, and he relished the ability to check his intensity levels during exercise with a heart rate monitor. "I'm a numbers kind of guy, so having

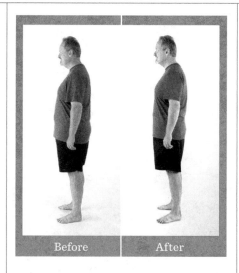

Before | After

that automatic feedback really helped me to figure out if I was exercising at about the right intensity." He also discovered that his previous cardio workouts (which often included some leisurely reading while he pedaled) were far too easy. He switched from the stationary bike to a treadmill at the gym, and he says having to keep up with the machine kept him in line.

Trying out a variety of new strength moves also made a big difference in his fitness. "I discovered that while I was doing a lot of resistance exercises, they weren't necessarily the right kind. This plan worked my muscles in a whole new way, and I wasn't as strong as I thought—I was actually shocked at how weak I really was!" He saw some of the biggest improvements in both his upper-body strength and his balance.

It's not uncommon for men to lose

weight more quickly than women, and for Burt the pounds came off fast. He lost about 5 pounds in his first week, a bit more in his second, and then another 8 pounds or so in his third week on the plan. As a person with type 2 diabetes, Burt had to follow his own dietary guidelines, but he found that simply keeping an eye on his portions and eating regular meals and snacks paid off.

In addition to some of the outward changes—in just 4 weeks he dropped 3 inches from his waist, bringing his pants size from a 44 to a 41, and another 2 inches off his hips—Burt's been able to gain some control over his diabetes. "Thanks to the weight loss I've experienced on the plan, my doctor said I could reduce my diabetes medication. Now I just have to keep up my end of the exercise and diet regimen."

While he's very pleased with his weight loss, he says he's not done yet. "I haven't weighed this number since my son was born—and he's now 25!" Burt's ultimate goal is to get down to about 200 pounds or less, which he plans to reach by keeping up with the strength and cardio workouts. "I've had great success from the start, and now I'm motivated to keep it up."

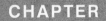

CHAPTER

4

Getting On Board: A Transition Week

If you haven't been working out regularly, starting a new fitness program can be a bit intimidating. It's kind of like asking someone who's been out of school for 15 years to start doing calculus or someone who hasn't played piano since she was a kid to run through a sonata.

So before you get ready to begin the 4-week Turn Up Your Fat Burn program, consider taking the next week to prepare yourself, both physically and mentally, with our "on-board" program. Think of it as the on-ramp to your superhealthy highway, a chance to gradually accelerate your fitness levels, eating habits, and emotional relationship with activity and to help your muscles—and your mind—start to move in the right direction.

The prep week is an opportunity to get ready for action, so you're not going from zero to sixty when you start the full program. It's a great way for you to start taking ownership of your program and prepare for the challenges ahead.

The on-board week includes some basic stretching, strength activities, and cardio. Use this week to help you figure out the logistics of regular physical activity. What's the best time of day for you to exercise? What do you need to eat before and after so you feel energized but not overly stuffed? What equipment do you need to help you perform at your best? How should you feel during and after a workout?

We put together this simple program to gradually introduce your muscles to weight training and start to build your cardiovascular base. For this on-board week, do the stretching and strength series together at least 2 days (give yourself at least 1 rest day in between so your muscles have time to recover). Begin with the warmup and dynamic stretching series, which is designed to get your muscles and joints ready for the strength moves. In addition, try to do two or three 20- to 30-minute aerobic workouts at a moderate intensity (RPE of 5 or 6), whether that's going for a bike ride or taking a brisk walk. And don't forget to check out the food basics in the previous chapter, which will help you get a handle on how your eating habits may be changing during the program (and, hopefully, from here on out!).

WHO SHOULD GET ON BOARD?

If you haven't been active regularly—say, working out at least 3 or 4 days a week for the past 3 months, with some form of strength training at least 2 of those days—it's a good idea to do the on-board week. Following it for even just a few days will make a big difference in reducing muscle soreness and getting you used to the program.

Most of our panel participants who did the on-board week were happy they did so, because it helped them transition to the full 4-week plan. "It definitely helped me jump-start my program," notes Kimberly Hampsey. "I was really glad that I did the on-board week," adds Leslie Kingston. "The transition into the full program the following week was so much easier!"

If you haven't been active recently (or ever!) or if you simply want a refresher, the preplan strength routine can get you familiar with some of the movement patterns you'll be doing over the following month. It can also help reduce some of the early muscle soreness that can occur with exercising after being inactive. The cardio program also helps reduce soreness and gets you up and moving so you're not in for a major shock when the full plan begins.

If you are already exercising regularly, congrats! You can start the full Turn Up Your Fat Burn program as soon as you are ready to get the body-changing results you've been seeking. Begin by taking the VT1 test in Chapter 5 to find your perfect training zone. Then move on to Week 1 of the full 4-week plan in Chapter 6.

WARMUP AND DYNAMIC STRETCHES

Warmup: March or jog in place or go for a walk at a comfortable pace for 3 to 5 minutes. You should be able to maintain a conversation easily, but go fast enough that it doesn't feel like you're window shopping.

Then do the following dynamic stretches for about 30 seconds each, moving at your own pace. Keep the movements under control.

1 Knee Lift

Walk or march forward or in place, bringing your lifted knee to your chest. Try twisting gently to the opposite direction as you move (so if you're lifting your right leg, bring it toward the left as your torso twists to the right). Alternate sides.

Butt Kicks

Walk or jog in place, bending your knees
to bring your heels toward your butt.

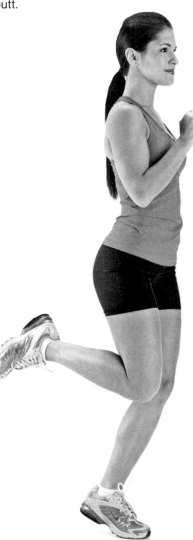

③ Frankenstein Walk

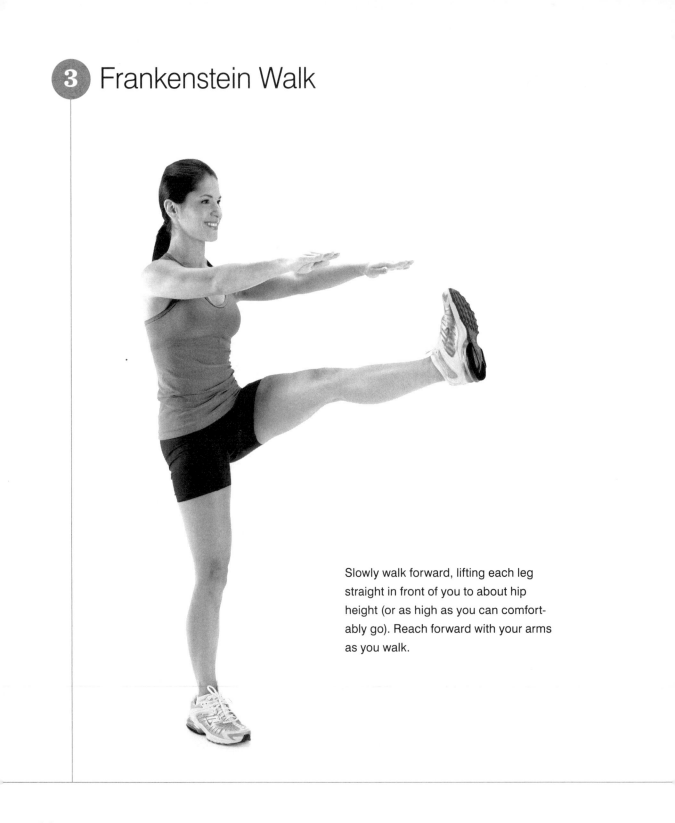

Slowly walk forward, lifting each leg straight in front of you to about hip height (or as high as you can comfortably go). Reach forward with your arms as you walk.

④ Cat-Back Stretch

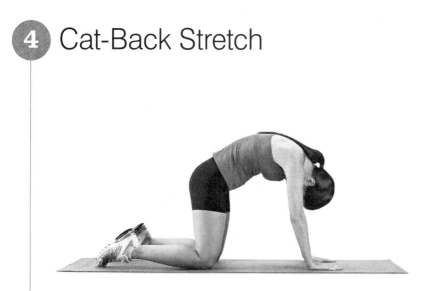

a. Begin on your hands and knees. Round your back, contracting your abdominals and tucking your pelvis under.

b. Reverse the movement and arch your back like a cat, lifting your tailbone up and your chest forward while raising your head. Repeat the rounding and arching motions for 30 seconds.

⑤ Chest/Back Stretch

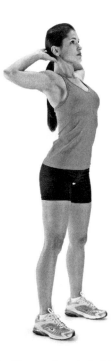

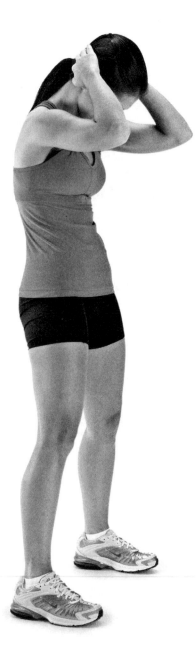

a. Stand with your hands behind your head, elbows out to the sides. Gently pull your elbows back as far as you comfortably can, arching your spine as you lift your chin, gazing up and feeling the stretch along your chest.

b. Keeping your hands where they are, bring your elbows together in front of your face, rounding your back and dropping your chin toward your chest, feeling the stretch along your upper back. Repeat the arching and rounding motions for 30 seconds.

ON-BOARD STRENGTH WORKOUT

After you've warmed up with the stretches, it's time for the strength circuit. Do **one full circuit** of all the following moves in the order given. Try to keep the rest time between exercises to a minimum—no more than 15 to 20 seconds. This will keep your heart rate elevated and prepare you for the more advanced circuit training in the month ahead. The full circuit should take about 20 minutes. Do this routine twice this week, giving yourself at least 48 hours between workouts.

What you'll need: A bench or sturdy low chair and a set of light weights. You can also use some everyday items to provide resistance if you don't have weights this week—see page 47 for more info on subbing household items for weights.

Finding the Perfect Weight

It's tempting to simply pick up any old dumbbell and start hoisting away, but to get the most out of your strength routine, it's important to choose a weight that's right for you. Think like Goldilocks: not too light, or you'll be using more momentum than muscle power. Not too heavy, or you may poop out too early to get results (or, even worse, risk injury). The perfect weight is one that's just right: heavy enough so you feel like you've really worked your target muscles by the final repetition, light enough that you can get through all the suggested reps without having to cheat or use additional muscles (for example, using your hips or back to push through an arm exercise).

Take the time during this on-board week to experiment and find the weights that are right for you. If you feel like you can breeze through 20 reps at the end of a set, you need to step it up on your next set or circuit. On the other hand, if you're struggling to get to even 8 reps, try lowering the weight (or in some cases use just your body weight). Finally, remember there's no such thing as a one-weight-fits-all workout. Bigger muscle groups can handle bigger loads, so the weight you're using for an arm or shoulder exercise would not be suitable for a chest, back, butt, or leg move. Try going up at least one weight size for exercises that target these larger body parts.

1 Bodyweight Squat

(works: legs, glutes)

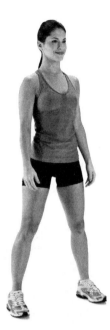

a. Stand with your feet a little more than hip-distance apart, hands at your sides.

b. Bend your knees about 90 degrees (or as far as you can) as if sitting in a chair, concentrating on keeping your weight over your heels (you should be able to see your toes if you look down). Bring your arms in front of you, elbows bent and hands at chest height, to help counterbalance the movement. Stand up and return to the starting position. Do as many repetitions as you can with good form until you feel fatigued.

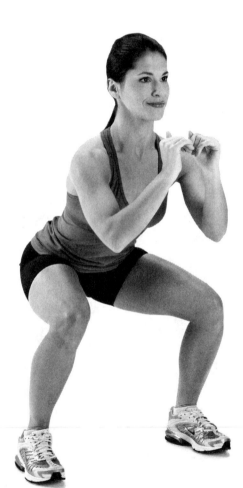

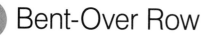

② Bent-Over Row

(works: upper back)

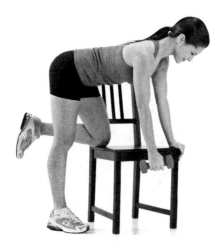

a. Stand to the right side of a sturdy low chair or low bench, holding a weight in your right hand. Place your left knee and left hand on the chair, and keep your right arm straight, with your hand under your shoulder.

b. Draw your right elbow up toward your ribs, keeping your arm close to your body, until the weight is about even with your ribs. Lower and repeat for 10 to 12 reps; switch sides.

FORM TIP! Keep your abdominal muscles engaged to stabilize your trunk, and avoid rotating your core during the row.

③ Step-Up and Hold

(works: legs, glutes)

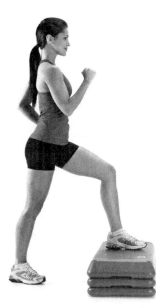

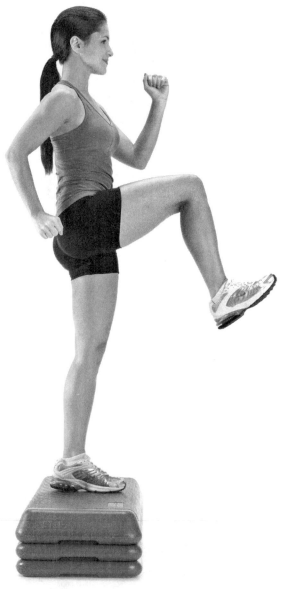

a. Stand facing a low bench or sturdy low chair, your arms at your sides with your elbows bent. Place your left foot on the bench or chair.

b. Step up, lifting your right knee toward your chest and bringing your left arm forward and right arm back. Avoid bending at the waist; keep your back straight. Hold for one count. Slowly step your right foot back to the floor, then your left foot. Repeat, placing your right foot on the bench and lifting your left leg. Do 10 to 12 reps per side, alternating legs.

④ Standing Torso Twist
(works: obliques)

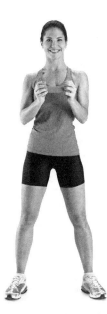

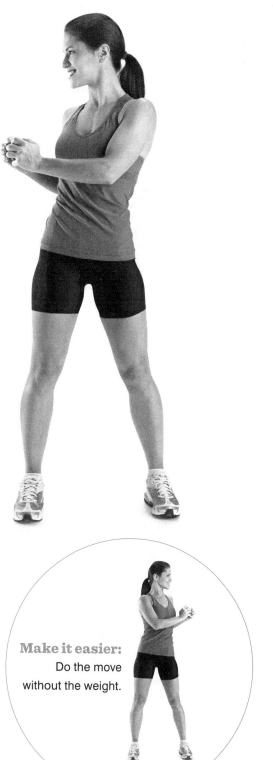

a. Stand with your feet 6 to 12 inches apart. Hold a light weight with both hands in front of your chest.

b. Rotate your upper body and head to the right as far as possible, holding for a moment without bouncing, then rotate back to the center. Repeat, rotating to the left and back to center. Continue rotating right and left, keeping your lower body still and your hips facing forward. Do 15 to 20 rotations per side.

Make it easier: Do the move without the weight.

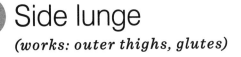

⑤ Side lunge

(works: outer thighs, glutes)

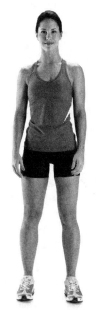

a. Stand with your feet hip-distance apart, your arms at your sides. Engage your abs.

b. Step your left foot out to the left side, keeping your weight over your heels and both feet facing forward. Shift your hips back, bending the left knee 90 degrees; keep your knee aligned between the second and third toes of your left foot and your shin perpendicular to the floor. (Your right leg is straight, with most of your weight shifted to your left hip.) Step back to start. Repeat, stepping your right foot out to the right side. Do 10 to 12 reps per side.

6 Seated overhead press

(works: shoulders)

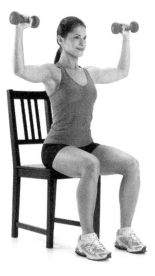

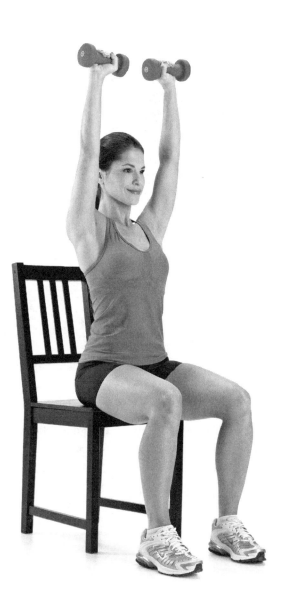

a. Sit holding light weights, with your elbows bent 90 degrees at shoulder height and palms facing forward.

b. Straighten your arms, bringing the weights overhead. Lower your elbows back to shoulder height and repeat. Do 10 to 12 reps.

FORM TIP! Keep your core muscles engaged and avoid arching your lower back during the press.

Pushup

(works: chest, arms, abs)

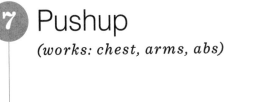

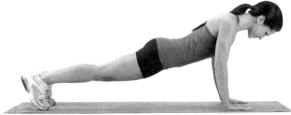

a. Begin in a full pushup position, your hands on the floor and your legs extended behind you. Shift your weight forward so your shoulders are over your hands; contract your abs.

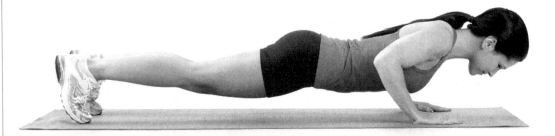

b. Slowly lower your body toward the floor, bending your elbows so your arms flare out slightly. Press back up to the starting position. Do 10 to 12 reps.

Make it easier:
Do a modified pushup with your knees on the floor.

8 Swimmer

(works: back)

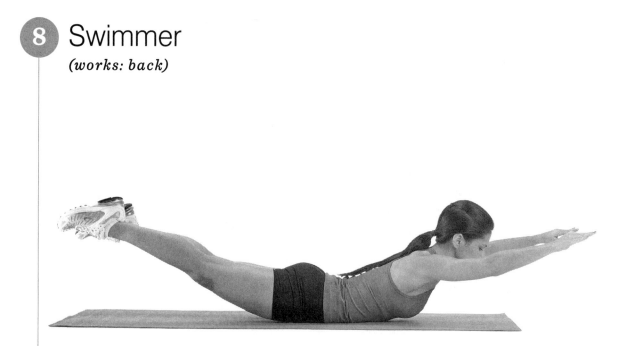

Lie facedown on the floor, your arms and legs
outstretched. Lift your arms, head, and chest
a few inches off the floor; then lift your legs.
Hold for 5 to 10 seconds, keeping your upper
body and legs lifted, then lower and repeat.
Do 3 to 5 repetitions.

⑨ Bridge

(works: hamstrings, glutes)

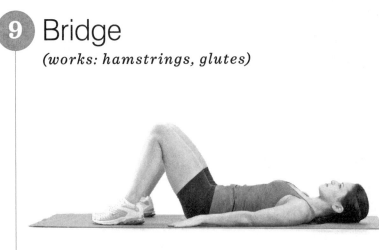

a. Lie faceup on the floor with your knees bent, heels on the floor, and arms next to your sides with palms down.

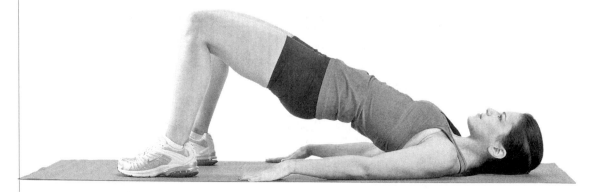

b. Engage your abs to flatten your lower back and lift your hips, keeping your abs tight. Hold for one count, then lower to the starting position and repeat. Do 15 to 20 reps.

10 Triceps Dip
(works: triceps)

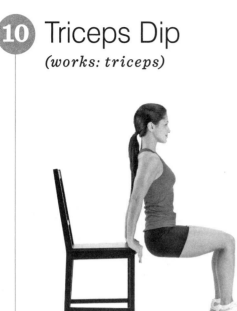

a. Sit on the edge of a sturdy chair or bench, your hands at the edge of the seat with your fingers facing forward. Keep your knees bent and your feet on the floor. Lift your hips off the bench and walk your feet a couple of inches forward, keeping your knees over your ankles.

b. Lower your butt toward the floor, bending your elbows directly behind you. Straighten your arms and repeat the dip, keeping your body close to the chair or bench. Do 10 to 12 reps.

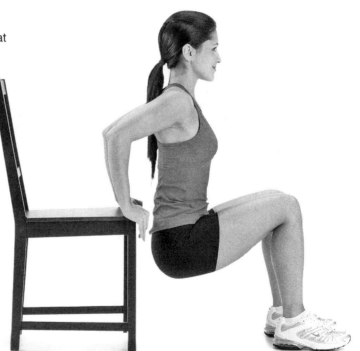

(11) Plank

(works: abdominals)

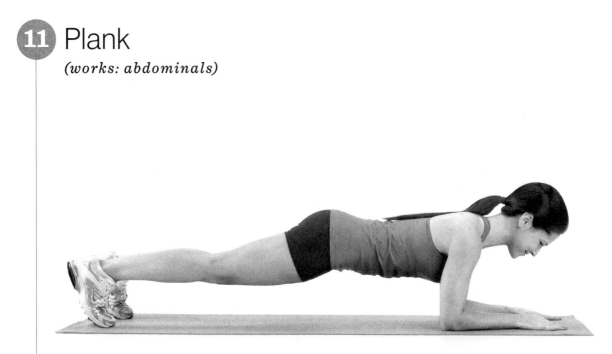

Lie facedown on the floor, your elbows under
your shoulders with your forearms on the
floor, fingers facing forward and legs
extended behind you, feet about hip-distance
apart. Lift your hips, forming a straight line
from head to heels and keeping your abs
tight. Hold for 20 to 60 seconds.

Make it easier:
Do this exercise in a full
pushup position, your arms straight
with your palms on the floor directly
beneath your shoulders.

STATIC STRETCHES

Finish your strength workout with a few static stretches to help increase your range of motion and speed your muscle recovery. Hold each stretch for about 15 to 30 seconds.

1 Hamstrings Stretch

a. Stand with your legs together, then extend your right leg with your heel on the ground. Bend your left knee slightly.

b. Reach forward and grasp your right ankle or shin, keeping your right leg straight. Stretch your hamstrings and lower back by gently pulling toward your leg.

2 Standing Quad Stretch

a. Support yourself by lightly holding onto a wall or chair with your left hand. Bend your right knee, grabbing your ankle behind you.

b. Gently pull your foot toward your butt; hold for 15 to 30 seconds, relax, and repeat on the opposite leg.

3 Calf Stretch

a. Stand facing a wall about 12 inches away from you. Take a big step behind you with your right foot, keeping both feet on floor and bending your left knee.

b. Lean into the wall, feeling tension along the right calf muscle. Hold for 15 to 30 seconds; switch sides and repeat.

4 Shoulder Stretch

a. Extend your right arm across your chest, your palm facing your body.

b. Gently pull your right forearm toward your body with your left forearm, feeling the stretch along the outside of your right shoulder. Hold for 15 to 30 seconds; switch sides and repeat.

5 Upper-Back/Chest Stretch

a. Interlace your fingers and extend your arms out in front, palms facing your body.

b. Drop your head and round your upper back; hold for 15 to 30 seconds.

c. Reverse the stretch, grasping your hands together behind you, palms facing your body; look up, arching your spine.

ON-BOARD CARDIO WORKOUT

Having an aerobics "base" on which to build can make a big difference in turning you into a more efficient exerciser. It usually takes several weeks to build a base. But even if you haven't been doing any regular aerobic exercise, you can still use this week as a starting point to get your body used to the activity and determine the right intensity level for your 4-week exercise program. Intensity is key to getting results in the Turn Up Your Fat Burn plan. Figuring out if you're working too hard (or not hard enough!) will help you make the most of every minute of your workout and turn you into a more efficient fat-burning machine.

Use Your RPE

As we mentioned in the last chapter, your rate of perceived exertion, or RPE, is a great way to gauge how hard you're working during exercise. Take this week to get a feel for different intensity levels and rate them as often as possible. What does it feel like at 3, 5, 8, or even 9? You probably won't have to push yourself all the way to 10, but imagine how it might feel to go to your max.

Recognizing these different exertion levels will be an important part of your 4-week program. Don't worry; we'll give you more guidelines to help you along. This week we just want you to get used to differences in intensity levels.

Commit to two or three 20- to 30-minute cardio workouts

Each workout should feel hard enough that you're somewhat breathless, but not so hard that you couldn't keep it up for the full time.

Add a little time or intensity to each session. This will prepare you for the cardio program in the 4-week plan, which incorporates 2 or 3 days of cardio for 25 to 35 minutes. But don't add too much or go out too hard—remember, this is your on-board week, designed to prepare you for the workouts to come.

Understand your cardio goals

Your goal is to add 5 to 10 percent to your "training volume" for each workout. Training volume is calculated by multiplying time by intensity. For example, if you plan to do 20 minutes of cardio at an RPE of 5 on Monday, your total training volume for that session will be 100 (20×5).

In your next workout (let's say on Wednesday), boost that number to 105 to 110. You could choose to go a little longer (22 minutes at an RPE of 5 $(22 \times 5 = 110)$ or work a little harder $(20 \times 5.5 = 110)$.

If you plan to complete a third cardio workout this week (let's say on Saturday), increase your volume once again by 5 to 10 percent. Now 105 to 110 becomes 115 to 121. That may mean going a little longer (23 minutes $\times 5 = 115$) or boosting your RPE again (20 minutes $\times 6 = 120$).

Why all the math? It's important to build up your exercise program gradually so you're not doing too much too soon. When you challenge yourself slowly but steadily, you'll continue to see improvements in fitness and in weight loss. You can increase the intensity (how hard an exercise feels), frequency (how often you exercise), or duration (how long you exercise). The formula above includes all three components, so you can safely raise your fitness level while seeing real results.

We want this week (and the next month—not to mention the rest of your life!) to be a thoroughly positive experience. So, while our program gives you the flexibility to set your own duration and intensity, don't push too hard or beyond what you predict is manageable.

MARIXSA ALI

Age: 39

Height: 5'2"

Pounds lost: 10

Inches lost: 3¾

What she's most proud of: "Being a good role model for my family."

Favorite foods: Tuna with mayo and boiled green bananas; low-fat yogurt and fruit

Like many people, when Marixsa Ali decided she needed to lose weight, she joined a local gym. But instead of easing into a regular routine, she went full blast, and soon her all-or-nothing attitude got her into trouble. "I got up at 5:30 in the morning and did the treadmill, then went back again after work and did some more cardio," she recalls. After a couple of months, the stress took its toll, and she tore part of her Achilles tendon, making almost any form of exercise too painful.

After a few months of inactivity, Marixsa says she hit more than 200 pounds. She started riding a stationary bike at home and walking on her lunch hour, and soon she started to lose weight but felt she needed more structure. "I wanted to follow a plan that would get me on a regular routine," she says.

Marixsa also wanted to set a good

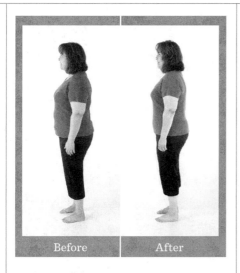

Before | After

example for her youngest daughter, who at 10 is starting to battle her own weight problems. "When you're a parent who has made the wrong food choices over and over again, you have to address your own decisions before you can help your children. I can't expect her to eat right and exercise if I'm not doing the same."

Battling a busy schedule (in addition to her job in sales at a local newspaper, Marixsa is going back to school for nursing and helping to raise her 4-month-old granddaughter, who also lives with her) meant having a workout program that was regimented but also efficient. She often squeezes in an exercise session between dropping her daughter off at the school bus stop and going to work or when she first gets home at night. "I put on my exercise clothes immediately, so I get into the

right frame of mind. If I'm already wearing what I'm going to work out in, I know I'll do it."

And while most of her past workouts focused on cardio, Marixsa says she likes the variety and the results that strength training brings. "I usually just try to do some walking or biking, but incorporating the weights has made a big difference," she reports. During her 4 weeks on the panel, she lost 10 pounds and 2 inches off her waist, as well as an inch off her hips.

After finishing the official program, Marixsa was determined to keep going. "My clothes are a little looser now, but I'm not done yet—I'm going on vacation to Puerto Rico at the end of the year, and I want to be down at least one more size," she reported.

Five months after starting the program, Marixsa is down 22 pounds. "I'm still trying to choose healthier options at the grocery store for myself and my family. I've been super busy, but I make an effort to get the workouts in whenever I can. There are moments when I think twice about exercising, but I'm committed. My overall goal is to eventually lose 40 more pounds, and I know I'm well on my way."

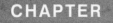

CHAPTER 5

Finding Your Fat-Burning Sweet Spot

There's just one more thing you need to do before you dive into the Turn Up Your Fat Burn plan, and that's determine your Ventilatory Threshold 1 (VT1), your fat-blasting sweet spot.

Everyone has a personal VT1 level. A world-class marathoner might be able to run a 7-minute mile and easily chat with her running buddy, while someone who hasn't run for more than shelter during a rainstorm might be gasping for breath when walking a 15-minute mile. No matter where you are now, with the right training, you can bump your VT1 to a higher level. What makes you breathless today can seem easy breezy in just a few weeks.

Our aim is train your body to work at ever-higher levels so you burn more calories each minute, while keeping you in a high fat-burning zone. Since most of us are exercising more for health (okay, and a sleeker physique) than to be medal contenders, the more efficiently we burn fat, the closer we will be to reaching our better-body goals.

For most of the cardio workouts in your 4-week plan, you'll be training in and around the magical VT1 threshold. But just how do you determine your unique zone? This chapter will help you test whether you are exercising at the right intensity, not too fast and not too slow. It's about finding what's just right, and it's easier than you may think.

THE TALK TEST

The talk test is a well-regarded measure of exercise intensity. It's as simple as it sounds. You can fairly objectively determine how easy or hard you are exercising by how many words you can say without having to pause to take a breath. The talk test has been used for years by trainers and fitness pros to customize exercise intensity.

If while exercising you can go into full detail about the latest escapades in your office or go on a long rant about some family drama, you're probably moving at a low intensity. The harder you work, the more difficult it is to breeze through a conversation. If you increase your intensity to a moderately high rate, you can string together a few words or a short sentence without having to take a breath. Go at an all-out sprint and you probably won't be able to blurt out more than a syllable or two at a time. You also won't be able to keep up this intensity for very long.

Research shows that the talk test is closely tied to how fast your heart is beating and how much oxygen you are utilizing during exercise. The talk test also ties neatly into VT1.

At VT1, your body shifts from burning fat as your main fuel to burning more carbs. When your body is burning mostly fat, which for most of us is the primary goal, you can still speak fairly evenly and clearly.

You can string together a couple of sentences and talk continuously for several seconds. In reality, that means you can give a chuckle about Jon Stewart's latest take on *The Daily Show* or rehash the latest *Saturday Night Live* digital short with maybe a little huffing and puffing. At this level, you require more oxygen to burn the fat, but you're exhaling relatively little carbon dioxide. It's during the exhale that we talk, so your ability to speak isn't compromised. (Ever try talking while inhaling? Not easy.)

When you increase intensity with more speed or resistance (like an incline on a treadmill), you can still chat but can get out only a couple of short phrases at a time. Your cardiovascular system brings in more oxygen so your working muscles can do their thing. Your lungs have to push out the increased by-product of this respiratory process, carbon dioxide. You're breathing faster, and the more breaths you have to take, the harder it is to speak coherently.

That's why the talk test works so well for determining your VT1: It allows you to measure the point at which your body shifts from burning more fat to burning more carbs!

USING RPE

The rate of perceived exertion, or RPE, introduced in Chapter 4, goes hand in hand with the talk test. RPE is another important way to determine your intensity during exercise. To recap, RPE ranks exertion on a scale of 1 to 10, with 1 being oh-so-easy (we're talking feet-up-on-the-couch territory) and 10 your absolutely maximum effort (sprinting-to-catch-a-plane hard).

Combining RPE and the talk test can help you figure out whether you should be walking or running a little faster, using a wee bit more resistance on a machine like a stationary bike or elliptical trainer, or increasing the incline a tad on the treadmill.

Just How Hard Are You Working?

INTENSITY	RPE	FEELS LIKE	TALK TEST
No effort	1–2	Watching TV on the couch	Easy conversation
Very light	3	Window shopping	Easy conversation
Light	4	Walking to get somewhere	Very slightly breathless (mostly sentences)
Moderate	5	Walking to an appointment for which you're a little late	Slightly breathless (short sentences/phrases)
Moderately hard	6	Walking to cross the street before the light changes	Somewhat breathless (short phrases)
Somewhat vigorous	7	Late for a meeting with your boss/late for school pickup	Noticeably breathless (a few words at a time)
Vigorous	8	Very late for a meeting with your boss/very late for pickup	Noticeably breathless (a few words with difficulty)
Very vigorous	9	Late for a plane/running to get somewhere	Very breathless (hard to speak more than a word or two)
All-out effort	10	Sprinting to catch your plane	Can't speak

MONITORING YOUR HEART RATE

For years, athletes have used heart rate monitors in training. The monitor is usually worn on a chest strap just above the bra line for women and around the chest for men. There's also an accompanying wristwatch. The device is like a little window into your heart. It tells you how many times your heart is beating each minute, indicating how hard you're working. By comparing this number to your maximum heart rate, you have a completely objective sense of whether you're working too hard or not hard enough.

Today you can find a basic heart rate monitor for under $50 online and at sporting goods stores, as well as at mass merchandisers like

Cardio machines have come a long way from the nonmotorized, self-powered devices that required quite a bit of work on your part just to get the wheels turning. Today you can find an aerobic training tool to mirror almost any movement out there (and maybe a few you hadn't even thought of). From treadmills, stationary bikes, and stairclimbers to elliptical trainers, rowers, arcs, and skating machines, there's a piece of cardio equipment to match every taste, preference, and style. Many are loaded with bells and whistles, from fans to cool you off to video games where you race against a computerized opponent to keep you motivated.

If you're not wearing a heart rate monitor around your chest, many machines will allow you to check in and track your heart rate while you're exercising. A built-in monitor will keep track of your pulse as you grip the handlebars for brief periods. While these pulse monitors can provide some objective sense of how hard you are working, they are notorious for being extremely inaccurate. In fact, you can sometimes set one off when you're not even touching it. There can also be a significant delay between your actual heart rate and the reading on the monitor, so you might be working at a number as high as 175 but see a readout that's a dozen points lower because the machine hasn't yet caught up.

Going by the principle that something is better than nothing, if you don't have a heart rate monitor and you do have access to a machine like a treadmill with a built-in pulse monitor, take note of the readout on the console, along with your own rate of perceived exertion when you take the VT1 test. This way you can at least use those numbers as a guide to help you determine your RPE during future training.

Target or Walmart. Many trainers and coaches consider the heart rate monitor one of the greatest fitness inventions of the last 20 years.

If you've worked with a trainer or been to a gym, you may have experienced zone training based on percentage of maximum heart rate. At a relatively low level of intensity (about 50 to 60 percent of your maximum heart rate), you may find it easy to talk, and your exertion may be only 3 or 4 on a scale of 1 to 10. As you increase intensity, your heart rate rises, as does your rate of perceived exertion, while your ability to speak becomes more and more difficult. At the highest zone (above 90 percent max heart rate), you may find it difficult to speak at all.

It sounds great, but how do you determine your maximum heart rate? Most formulas are too generic or simply too imprecise to help the average exerciser find his or her maximal rate. The most common formula, 220 minus your age, has been proven wildly inaccurate, because individual heart rates vary significantly among people of the same age. The results of this formula can be off by as many as 36 beats per minute. For a 30-year-old, the standard formula says the standard max heart rate is 190 beats per minute (220 – 30), but actually, it could be anywhere from 154 to 226 beats per minute.

VT training doesn't use heart rate to measure intensity, because it's more about breath rate than the number of times your heart beats per minute. So why bother with a heart rate monitor at all? The value lies in the objective measure of exercise intensity. Although RPE and the talk test offer insights into your intensity level, they are based on your own opinion of when an exercise feels challenging. A monitor offers an unbiased guide to intensity—the numbers don't lie. Having a set number to put with your talk test and perceived intensity can make it a little easier to determine your VT1 number, which will allow you to develop a more precise and effective training program. "I learned a lot about my intensity levels when I had the heart rate monitor on," reports panelist Cindy Wenrich. "Having a hard number to put with my effort level gave me a better sense of just how hard I really was working and where I needed to be."

DETERMINING YOUR VT1

Now that we've introduced some of the tools and guidelines, it's time to figure out your own VT1. One important note: Your VT1 can vary depending on the activity performed; some types of exercise are higher impact than others, plus you use different muscles and have a different center of gravity, all of which can affect your VT1. That means the number you get on the treadmill could be different from the one on the stationary bike, in part because on the treadmill, more of your upper body gets in on the action. You can still use different types of cardio during training, but for this test, choose the type of workout you think you will use most often during the next 4 weeks.

Your goal is to determine at what pace or intensity level you can no longer comfortably talk out loud without getting very breathless. So apologize in advance to the people around you if you work out in a public fitness facility, and get ready to go!

This entire test should take about 15 to 20 minutes. Ask a friend or training partner to write down the numbers you will be giving him or her. For best results, do the test twice, on two different days, and take an average of the results. (If you're planning to do the on-board program, this may also be a good time to practice the VT1 test.) This can help give you a better understanding of how to gradually increase your intensity and how your heart rate responds.

Step 1

Begin by warming up at a light effort for 3 to 5 minutes (RPE 3 to 4). This is your easy-conversation pace. If you're wearing a heart rate monitor, watch your heart rate level off, and stay there for at least a few minutes.

Step 2

Gradually increase your workload by small increments every couple of minutes (on a treadmill, increase each time by 0.5 mph or a 1 percent grade).

Feel good? Continue to increase the workload to a pace you feel you could maintain for a long period of time but makes you a little bit breathless. If you're wearing a heart rate monitor, watch for the number to level off, which should happen after about 30 to 60 seconds.

Here's the talking part of the test: Talk out loud for 20 to 30 seconds. You should be able to speak smoothly and continuously (not gasping for air but noticing when you have to take a breath).

Step 3

After the talk test, bump up the intensity slightly again, wait until your heart rate levels off, and repeat the talk test. Are you still able to speak smoothly and evenly? Continue to increase the intensity little by little, then repeat the talk test every couple of minutes, making sure your heart rate has leveled off each time before increasing the intensity.

Step 4

When speaking starts to become challenged (your words are choppy or forced out, but you're not gasping for air), you are at VT1.

If you're going to be training on the same machine throughout the program (and we recommend you do), keep note of your RPE and the speed and/or incline. If you're wearing a heart rate monitor, remember your BPM (beats per minute) at VT1.

Step 5

Continue to increase the intensity a few more times, increasing both RPE and breathing rate. Stay at each new level for at least 1 minute, allowing your heart rate to level off. Take note of your RPE, talk test results, and heart rate for each level. Stop when you get to the point when you can no longer say two or three words without having to take a breath.

It's important to keep going at least a little bit past your VT1 point so that you can have some idea of what it feels like to get more breathless during your intervals (and so you can avoid getting to this point in your weekly workouts on the program).

Step 6

Gradually start to cool down, until you are able to breathe easily and have an RPE of about 3 or 4.

Here's how this may play out for someone who is doing this test on a treadmill with 2-minute stages.

MINUTES	SPEED (MPH)/INCLINE (PERCENT)	TALK TEST	RPE (1–10)	HEART RATE
0–5	2.5/1	Easy conversation (warmup)	3–4	117
5–7	2.5/2	Easy conversation	4	125
7–9	3.0/2	Slightly breathless	5	133
9–11	3.5/2	A little more breathless but can still speak in sentences	6	138
11–13	4.0/2	Words are choppy or forced (VT1 as determined by talk test)	6½	142
13–15	4.5/3	Difficult to say more than a few words	7	147
15–16	5.0/3	Difficult to say more than 1 or 2 words	8–9	155
16–20	3.0/0	Cooldown	3	120

How you structure your VT1 test (incline, speed, type of machine, or no machine) is entirely up to you. Just determine the point at which your breathing becomes choppy. Don't worry if your VT1 seems low—you're going to be working a bit above this level in your intervals. On the other hand, be honest about what seems difficult or how difficult it may really be to speak. If your numbers are too low, you won't be challenging yourself enough during the intervals to make a difference in your fitness level and raise your VT1 or fat-burning level.

Write down your VT1 level so you'll have it handy when you are doing the cardio intervals during the plan.

VT1 Test

MINUTES	SPEED (MPH)/ INCLINE (PERCENT)	TALK TEST	RPE (1–10)	HEART RATE

SO HOW DO YOU REALLY FEEL?

Your workouts and eating habits aren't the only important aspects of the Turn Up Your Fat Burn program. Your emotional connection to fitness—how you feel about physical activity—also plays a key part in your overall success.

When you talk to someone who exercises regularly, he or she will invariably tell you that they can't imagine what it would be like to *not* work out at least several times a week. Exercise has become a healthy habit they can't live without.

Your workout experience—positive or negative—will significantly impact whether you continue to exercise long after you've finished the 4-week program. It's extremely important to leverage any good feelings you may have in the upcoming weeks. It may sound touchy-feely, but monitoring your emotional response to your workout experience—how you really feel about exercising—can make a big difference toward making you a lifelong exerciser.

Scientists use a simple tool called the Exercised-Induced Feeling Inventory (EFI) to measure emotional perceptions. Immediately following each workout the first week, take a few minutes to complete the following questionnaire. Continue to do so following each exercise session throughout the month.

Score each emotion according to how strongly you experience it after your workout. Record your response for each emotion by checking the appropriate number.

0 = Do not feel

1 = Feel slightly

2 = Feel moderately

3 = Feel strongly

4 = Feel very strongly

Add the scores for the words 4, 7, and 12. That's your score for positive engagement.

Add your scores for words 1, 6, and 9. That's your score for revitalization.

Add your scores for 2, 5, and 10. That's your score for tranquility.

Add your scores for 3, 8, and 11. That's your score for physical exhaustion.

Track your scores in each category over the next few weeks to keep tabs on changes in your emotions. If your average scores for physical exhaustion become smaller, for example, that means your energy levels are improving and you're probably feeling less fatigued after your workout. This type of information, tracked over time, provides excellent feedback on how your perceptions are changing toward your exercise experience. And the better you feel about exercise, the more likely you are to keep at it!

The opposite page shows how a typical log might play out. As you can see, over just 1 week, this exerciser has become increasingly more engaged during the workouts and feels more revitalized and tranquil—and less tired—afterward.

	STRENGTH WORKOUT 1	STRENGTH WORKOUT 2	CARDIO WORKOUT 1	CARDIO WORKOUT 2	CARDIO WORKOUT 3
Day/Date	Mon	Wed	Thurs	Fri	Sun
1. Refreshed	1	2	1	2	2
2. Calm	2	2	2	3	3
3. Fatigued	3	2	3	2	2
4. Enthusiastic	0	2	0	2	2
5. Relaxed	1	2	1	2	3
6. Energetic	0	2	1	2	3
7. Happy	1	1	2	3	3
8. Tired	3	2	3	2	1
9. Revived	1	2	1	2	2
10. Peaceful	1	2	1	2	2
11. Worn out	3	2	3	2	2
12. Upbeat	1	2	1	2	2
	TOTALS				
Positive engagement (4, 7, 12)	2	5	3	7	7
Revitalization (1, 6, 9)	2	6	3	6	7
Tranquility (2, 5, 10)	4	6	4	7	8
Physical exhaustion (3, 8, 11)	9	6	9	6	5

PART III

Turn Up Your Fat Burn: The Program

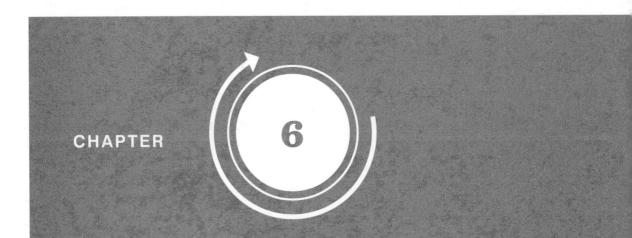

CHAPTER 6

Week 1

Time to put all of your new knowledge about maximizing fat loss to good use. Welcome to the first week of the Turn Up Your Fat Burn training plan. Get ready to do some work, break a sweat, and—most of all—have fun!

YOUR GOALS THIS WEEK

- Do two metabolic strength circuit workouts (about 30 to 40 minutes each).

- Do two fat-burning cardio interval workouts (about 30 minutes each).

- **Optional:** Do one moderate-pace cardio workout (about 30 minutes).

How you structure this program is entirely up to you. You can choose to do the strength and cardio on the same day or on different days. Just make sure you don't perform strength workouts on back-to-back days; you need to give your muscles time to recover and get stronger. You can add any other activities you like as long as you're still doing the prescribed cardio and strength workouts listed here.

Here's what a sample week might look like.

Monday: Metabolic strength circuit

Tuesday: Off

Wednesday: Cardio intervals

Thursday: Metabolic strength circuit

Friday: Off

Saturday: Cardio intervals

Sunday: Off or optional light cardio

And by the way, if you find that you're a little sore after your workouts, check out the advice on page 38.

How it works: Warm up by walking or jogging lightly for a few minutes and doing some dynamic stretching. Then start the strength circuit: Do the exercises in the order given, resting about 15 seconds between each move and a full 60 seconds at the end of the circuit. Complete the circuit three times. Do this workout two times this week on nonconsecutive days.

What you'll need: Light and medium weights, a sturdy chair or bench, and a mat (optional).

WARMUP AND STRETCH

March or jog in place or go for a walk at a comfortable pace for 3 to 5 minutes. You should be able to maintain an easy conversation, but go fast enough that it doesn't feel like you're out for a leisurely stroll.

Do the dynamic stretches starting on page 61 for about 30 seconds each, moving at your own pace. Keep the movements under control.

After the workout: Finish by doing the static stretches starting on page 75.

METABOLIC STRENGTH CIRCUIT

Week 1 This total-body strength circuit provides a strong foundation for your program. We're hitting all the major muscle groups here. Most of these exercises are fairly basic. If you've done the on-board week, you'll already be familiar with some of these moves. No matter if you didn't—you'll catch on quickly. You'll build upon each exercise as the program moves forward. For each exercise, use a weight that is heavy enough that your muscles feel like you've really worked them by the final rep.

So let's turn the page and get started!

1 Romanian Deadlift

(works: hamstrings, glutes)

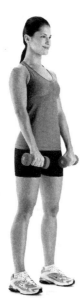

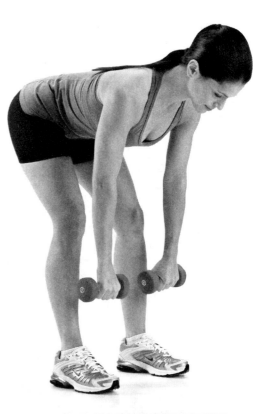

a. Stand with your feet hip-distance apart, holding medium weights in front of your thighs, palms facing your body.

b. Keeping your knees slightly bent and abs tight, hinge forward from your hips as you push your butt backward, slowly lowering the weights toward the floor. Squeeze your glutes as you stand back up. Repeat for a total of 12 to 15 reps.

FORM TIP! Make sure you feel the movement along the back of your legs (hamstrings), not in your lower back. Think of pushing your butt toward the wall behind you.

Chest Press

(works: chest, triceps, shoulders)

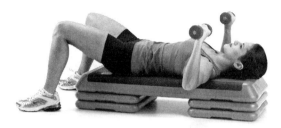

a. Lie faceup on a step or bench. (If you don't have either, lie on the floor and position a large pillow or sofa cushion vertically under your back.) Hold medium weights at chest level with your elbows bent and your palms forward with wrists neutral (not bent).

b. Straighten your arms and press the weights above your chest. Pause, then slowly lower the weights back toward your chest. Do 8 to 10 reps.

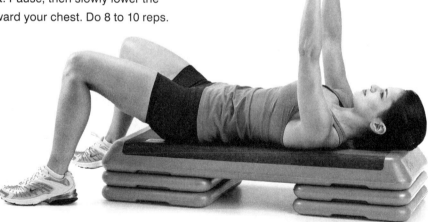

FORM TIP! Don't bring your elbows too far down as you lower the weight (they should stop at about the same height as your chest); exhale as you straighten your arms.

3 # Bent-Over Row
(works: upper back)

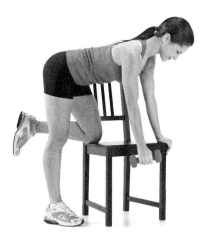

a. Place your left knee and left hand on a bench or sturdy low chair, holding a medium weight in your right hand with your arm extended directly under your shoulder. Keep your back flat and your head in line with your spine.

b. Draw your right elbow toward the sky, bringing the weight toward your ribs and keeping your arm close to your body. Continue to look down without arching your neck. Straighten your arm and repeat. Do 10 to 12 reps; switch arms and legs and repeat.

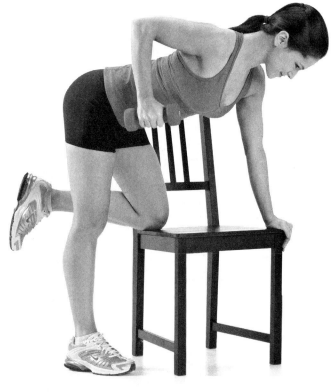

FORM TIP! Engage your abs by pulling in your belly button; keep your arm close to your body. You'll feel this more in your upper back than your arm.

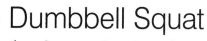

④ Dumbbell Squat

(works: quads, glutes)

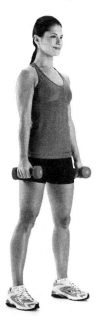

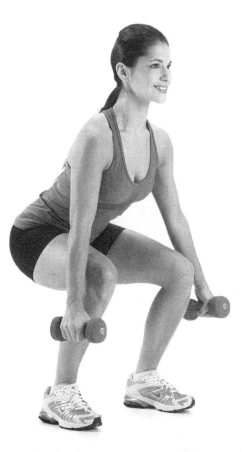

a. Stand with your feet hip-distance apart, holding medium weights at your sides.

b. Bend your knees about 90 degrees (or as far as you can) as if sitting in a chair. Stand up and return to the starting position. Do 10 to 12 reps.

FORM TIP! Keep your body weight over your heels and don't allow your knees to go too far forward—you should be able to see your toes if you look down.

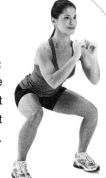

Make it easier:
Do this exercise without any weight (see bodyweight squat, Chapter 4).

⑤ Standing Shoulder Press

(works: shoulders)

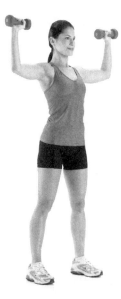

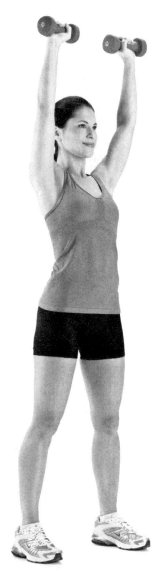

a. Stand with your feet a little wider than hip-distance apart, holding light or medium weights at shoulder height, your palms facing forward.

b. Straighten your arms and press the weights up, keeping your abs tight. Lower and repeat. Do 8 to 10 reps.

FORM TIP! Don't lock your elbows as you straighten your arms; try to keep your shoulders pressed down, not hunched up.

6 Stationary Lunge

(works: glutes, quads, hamstrings)

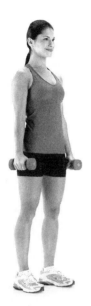

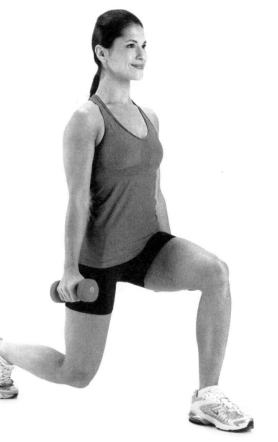

a. Stand with your feet hip-distance apart, holding medium weights at your sides, your palms facing your body.

b. Lunge your left leg forward, bending both knees 90 degrees and leaning forward slightly. Straighten your legs, keeping your feet planted, then bend your knees again. Do 12 to 15 reps. Switch sides and repeat.

FORM TIP! Keep your shoulders over your hips and your front knee directly above your ankle in the lunge; you should be able to see your toes if you look down.

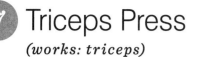

7 Triceps Press

(works: triceps)

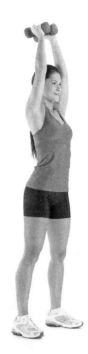

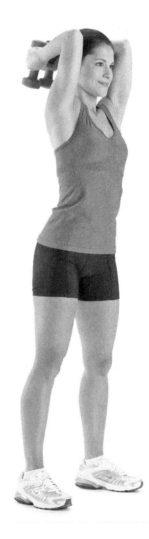

a. Hold two weights together above your head. (Option: Use just one slightly heavier weight.)

b. Bend your elbows and lower the weight behind your head. Straighten your arms and repeat. Do 8 to 10 reps.

FORM TIP! Keep your arms close to your ears as you lift and lower the weights.

8 Biceps Curl

(works: biceps)

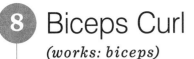

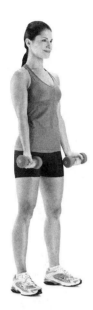

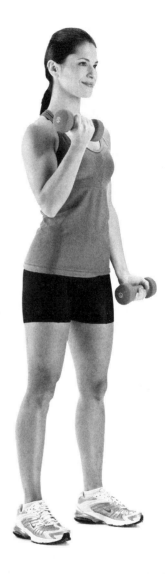

a. Stand tall with your arms at your sides, your palms facing forward as you hold light or medium weights.

b. Curl your right hand toward your right shoulder, then lower your right arm as you curl your left hand toward your left shoulder. Continue, alternating arms, for a total for 8 to 10 reps per side.

FORM TIP! Use a full range of motion as you lift and lower the weight; keep your arms close to your body.

9 Plié Squat

(works: glutes, quads, outer thighs)

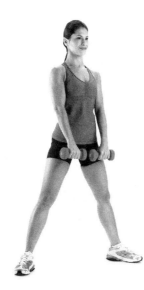

a. Stand with your feet just wider than shoulder-distance apart, toes turned out, holding medium weights in front of your thighs with your palms facing your body.

b. Pull in your abs to support your spine. Shift your hips back and down as you bend your knees 90 degrees, keeping your knees pointing in the same direction as your toes, your chest tall, and your abs tight. Squeeze your glutes as you return to the starting position. Repeat for 12 to 15 reps.

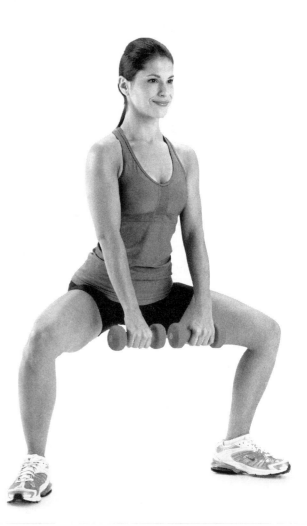

FORM TIP! Keep your knees tracking between your second and third toes; try not to allow the thighs to collapse inward.

10 Pushup

(works: chest, arms, abs)

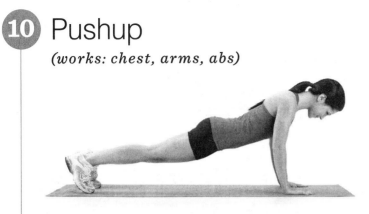

a. Begin in a full pushup position, your hands on the floor and your legs extended behind you. Contract your abs and shift your weight forward so your shoulders are over your hands.

b. Slowly lower your body toward the floor, bending your elbows so your arms flare out slightly. Press back up to the starting position. Do 10 to 12 reps.

FORM TIP! Don't let your hips sag as you come down toward the floor; contract your abs to help maintain your form. If pushups hurt your wrists, hold a pair of dumbbells on the floor to reduce some of the stress.

Make it easier:
Do a modified pushup with your knees on the floor.

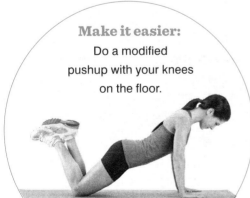

⓫ Plank

(works: abdominals, lower back)

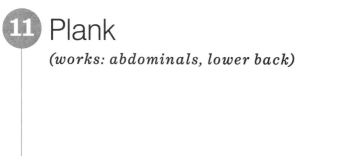

Lie facedown on the floor, your elbows under your shoulders with your forearms on the floor, fingers facing forward, and legs extended with your feet about hip-distance apart. Lift your hips, forming a straight line from head to heels, keeping your abs tight. Hold here for 20 to 60 seconds.

FORM TIP! Don't allow your hips to sink or arch back. Hold only as long as you can maintain good form; if you need to take a break, rest and then repeat.

Make it easier:
Do the move from a full pushup position, your arms straight with your palms on the floor directly beneath your shoulders.

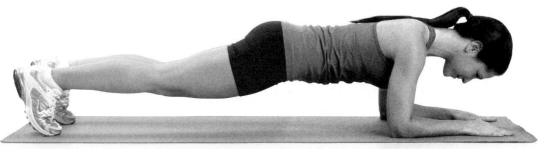

12 Bicycle

(works: abs, obliques)

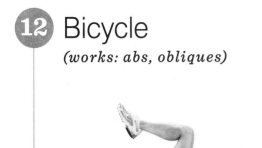

a. Lie faceup with your lower back pressed into the floor, your hands behind your head with your elbows out to the sides. Bring both knees toward your chest, lifting your head, neck, and shoulders off the floor.

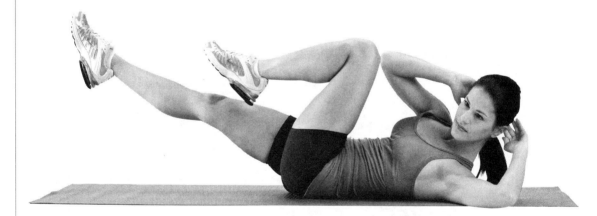

b. Lift your right shoulder toward your left knee while straightening your right leg. Switch sides, bringing your left shoulder toward your right knee. Continue for a total of 10 to 12 reps per side.

FORM TIP! Don't pull on your neck; think about bringing your shoulder rather than just the elbow toward the opposite knee.

FAT-BURNING CARDIO INTERVALS

Week 1

The Turn Up Your Fat Burn cardio plan includes 2 days each week of fat-burning intervals just above and below your VT1. Use the VT1 test in Chapter 5 as a guide. If you wore a heart rate monitor (or used a pulse monitor) during that test, try to keep the work portion of your cardio intervals about 10 beats higher than your VT1. (So if you were at 145 for the test, work at about 155 here.) You can also go by the talk test; during the interval portion, you should be breathing heavily but not so hard that you can't speak at all.

You can do any form of steady-state cardio (an activity that gradually increases your heart rate and intensity and keeps you there), but for best results, stick with the same type of workout that you did for your VT1 test. That's because your VT1 level riding a bike or working on the elliptical trainer will likely be different than when you are running. We happen to like the treadmill best—it gives precise control over your speed, provides more cushioning than many outdoor surfaces like asphalt or cement, and allows you to adjust the incline to increase intensity if you don't like to jog.

Do this workout twice this week, either on the same day as your metabolic strength circuit or on an alternate day. You can also add a third (optional) cardio workout: a steady-paced, moderate-intensity activity (RPE 5 to 6) like brisk walking or bicycling for about 30 minutes.

MINUTES	EFFORT	TALK TEST	HEART RATE (OPTIONAL)	RPE
0–3	Light (warmup)	Easy conversation	Below VT1	3–4
3–6	Medium-high	Challenging (short phrases)	10 beats above VT1	7
6–10	Medium	Easier (short sentences)	Just below VT1	5
10–13	Medium-high	Challenging (short phrases)	10 beats above VT1	7
13–17	Medium	Easier (short sentences)	Just below VT1	5
17–20	Medium-high	Challenging (short phrases)	10 beats above VT1	7
20–24	Medium	Easier (short sentences)	Just below VT1	5
24–25	Light (cooldown)	Easy (full conversation)	Below VT1	3–4

Excuse-Proof Your Workout

How many times have you started a regular exercise routine only to find yourself side-tracked? Here's how to reboot your attitude and get on the workout wagon for good!

THE EXCUSE: I DON'T HAVE TIME TO EXERCISE.
If you have time to watch TV, talk on the phone with a friend, or play around on the computer, you can find the time to squeeze in a workout. The secret is to find some holes in your schedule, even a few minutes. Take 10 minutes and go for a walk before breakfast, after lunch, and then again in the evening. Get up 30 minutes earlier tomorrow. When you have downtime on the weekend, go for a bike ride or find a place to hike with your family. Exercise isn't something you find time for. It's something you make time for.

THE EXCUSE: IT'S TOO HARD!
Don't give up now! One of the most rewarding parts of exercising is setting a goal and then achieving it. Think about what you'll be accomplishing when you exercise. It's not just about looking good, it's about feeling good today, tomorrow, and 10 years from now.

THE EXCUSE: I'M TOO TIRED AFTER A LONG DAY AT WORK TO EXERCISE.
The great thing about working out: Give a little, get a lot. Start out with just a few minutes—do one set of the strength moves, or just start the cardio routine. Odds are that once you get moving, you'll be more energized to continue. If you're still really too tired, get a good night's sleep and try switching your workouts to the morning for an all-day energy boost.

THE EXCUSE: I'M AFRAID I'LL GET HURT.
Starting with our on-board program will help ease you into the workouts so you're not as sore or achy. If you're still nervous about getting injured, keep your progressions slow. Stick to the Week 1 routine until you feel ready to move on. Invest in a good pair of athletic shoes to protect your muscles, joints, and ligaments while you work out. And remember: You'll be far healthier in the long run if you start to exercise today.

THE EXCUSE: I'M DESTINED TO BE HEAVY.
Genetics may play a role in your physique, but you hold the cards for how you will look, feel, and act. A recent British study of more than 20,000 people found that individuals with a high genetic predisposition to obesity were able to reduce their risks of becoming obese by an average of 40 percent just by being physically active.[1]

PAM GARIN

Age: 49

Height: 5'2"

Pounds lost: $8^{1}/_{2}$

Inches lost: $2^{1}/_{4}$

What she's most proud of: "I'm down at least one size and wearing things I haven't put on in year!"

Favorite foods: Quinoa mixed with brown rice and vegetables; whole wheat pretzels mixed with raisins

Like many former smokers, Pam Garin found herself exchanging food for cigarettes when she quit smoking 8 years ago. "The pounds just started rolling on," she says. The weight gain accelerated when Pam was in a car accident a couple of years ago, which left her with four herniated discs in her neck. Unable to do the exercise she loved the most—riding her bicycle with her husband—she watched the scale creep upward of 158 pounds.

"I just didn't feel healthy anymore," says Pam, despite losing (and regaining) weight through a series of diets. "I realized I was going to turn 50 soon, and I didn't want to be in the shape I was in." She set a goal for herself to drop a couple of sizes by her 50th birthday.

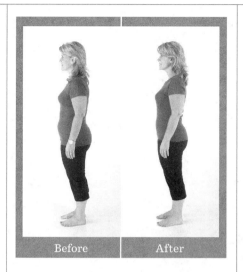

Before | After

Getting on the treadmill at 5:45 a.m. helped her squeeze in her cardio workouts and still have time to walk her Great Dane, Tulsa, before work. And while she never considered herself a runner, she says being able to jog the intervals on the treadmill has changed the way she looks at cardio. "Now when Tulsa and I go out, we don't just walk—we run!" she says, laughing.

But she credits the biggest changes to her strength-training program. "I hadn't picked up a weight in about 15 years, and I didn't realize that it could be such a good workout!" she says. Although her neck injury has kept her from doing some of the exercises, she's learned to modify moves so she can still get in a full workout.

Pam says that being able to stick to the modest diet guidelines is crucial. "I've changed everything about my eating habits," she notes. "I used to eat an early breakfast and wait until 3 p.m. to eat lunch, and by then I was totally starving. Now I pack everything the night before, so I have it when I need it." Her healthy habits have also influenced her family. "Before, when my husband and I went out to eat, I'd have just as big a serving as he was eating. Now we're splitting the main entrée and ordering extra vegetables as a side."

Her efforts paid off quickly: After 4 weeks on the plan, she'd lost 8½ pounds. But the biggest change has come in her confidence. "I put on one of my favorite red dresses, which I haven't worn in about 8 years, and it looked great! I even wore it with a belt, which I would never have dared to do before, because it would have drawn attention to my belly." She's even proudly pointing out the beginnings of a six-pack.

She's also noticed that exercise has given her a lot more energy to get through her often-12-hour workdays as the director of career services for a business school. And that big birthday that's right around the corner? It's not bothering her quite so much anymore: "I used to feel stiff just bending over to put my pants on, but now I actually feel younger when I wake up in the morning."

All of which has given her more incentive to keep at it. "This is just the start for me," says Pam. "I've gotten to a new place, and I'm not stopping now."

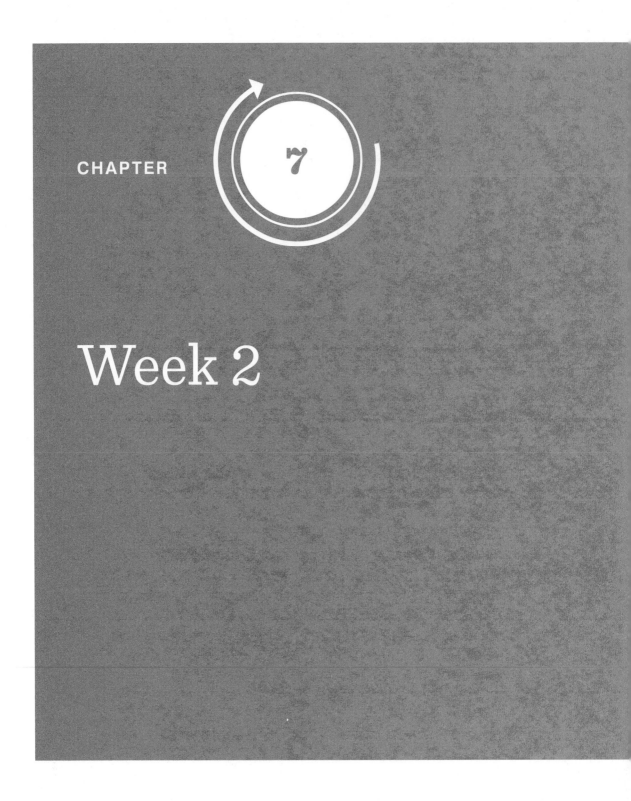

CHAPTER 7

Week 2

Welcome to Week 2! By now you should be feeling comfortable with the flow of the program and getting a feel for the routines. Hopefully, you're already starting to feel stronger and more energized. We'll continue this week with a menu of total-body workouts designed to make you leaner, fitter, and ready for action.

YOUR GOALS THIS WEEK

- Do two metabolic strength circuit workouts (two or three times through; about 35 to 45 minutes per session).
- Do two fat-burning cardio interval workouts (about 30 minutes each).
- **Optional:** Do one fat-burning cardio interval workout (about 30 minutes).

Here's what a sample week looks like:

Monday: Cardio intervals

Tuesday: Metabolic strength circuit

Wednesday: Off

Thursday: Metabolic strength circuit plus optional cardio intervals

Friday: Off

Saturday: Cardio intervals

Sunday: Optional additional activity (golf, hiking, cycling, etc.)

Warm up by walking for a few minutes and doing some dynamic stretching. Then start the strength circuit; complete this workout two times this week on nonconsecutive days.

WARMUP AND STRETCH

March or jog in place or go for a walk at a comfortable pace for 3 to 5 minutes. You should be able to maintain an easy conversation, but go fast enough that it doesn't feel like you're window shopping.

Then do the dynamic stretches starting on page 61 for about 30 seconds each, moving at your own pace. Keep the movements under control.

After the workout: Finish by doing the static stretches on page 75.

Go at Your Own Pace!

If you feel like you can't complete any of the exercises from this week's workout without keeping the right form, it's perfectly okay to repeat the moves from Week 1. When you're ready, try the moves designed for Week 2. It's better to do a basic exercise correctly than to do a more complex one wrong.

METABOLIC STRENGTH CIRCUIT

Week 2

This week we're building upon the exercises you learned last week, bringing the intensity up a notch. The moves are now a bit more challenging. You'll be working more muscles at the same time for a total-body workout that will boost your heart rate and give you a bigger postworkout afterburn. Stick with about the same weights you used for Week 1, but try to eke out two more reps for each exercise. If the dumbbells you chose last week felt too light, don't be afraid to challenge yourself a little and bump the weight up a bit.

This circuit takes a little longer and is more difficult; complete it at least twice, adding an optional third set depending on your time and energy level. Do the exercises in the order given, resting about 15 seconds between each move and a full 60 seconds at the end of the circuit.

What you'll need: Light and medium weights; a sturdy chair or bench; a paper plate, sheet of paper, or stability ball for the eighth move (bridge/hamstring curl); and a mat (optional).

So turn the page and let's get started!

1 Romanian Deadlift with Shoulder Press

(works: hamstrings, glutes, shoulders)

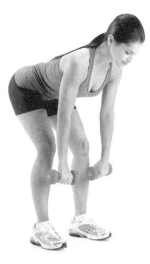

a. Stand with your feet hip-distance apart, holding medium or light weights in front of your thighs, palms facing your body. Keeping your knees slightly bent and abs tight, hinge forward from your hips as you push your butt backward. Slowly lower the weight toward the floor, pushing your butt straight back toward the opposite wall, keeping your knees slightly bent and abs tight.

b. Stand back up and bring the weights to shoulder height, your elbows bent and your palms facing forward.

c. (not shown) Straighten your arms, bringing the weights together overhead. Lower your elbows back to shoulder height, and then bring the weights in front of your thighs. Repeat the deadlift/press combo for 12 to 15 reps.

FORM TIP! Hinge forward from your waist to complete the deadlift; don't lock your knees. You should feel tension in your hamstrings. Pause for a moment after you stand up, then do the shoulder press.

② Pushup with Row

(works: chest, triceps, core, upper back)

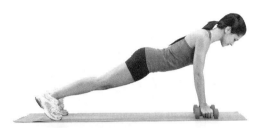

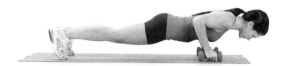

a. Begin in a full pushup position, hands holding light or medium weights on the floor under your shoulders and legs extended behind you, abs tight. Slowly lower your chest toward the floor, then straighten and repeat. Don't sink at the hips. Do 10 reps.

b. For the row, after your final rep, remain in the "up" position and lift your right hand, holding the weight. Bend your elbow, keeping your arm close to your body, lifting the weight until it's about even with your ribs. Lower and repeat. Do 8 to 10 reps, switch hands, and repeat.

FORM TIP! Remember to do all of the pushups first, then do the rows. During the rows, bring your feet wider apart to help keep you stable.

Make it easier:
Do a modified pushup with your knees on the floor. If this is still too difficult, you can do the pushup with your feet on the floor and your hands on a low counter or bench and do the row separately.

③ Alternating Lunge and Twist

(works: quads, glutes, obliques)

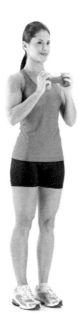

a. Stand tall, holding a medium weight horizontally in both hands close to your chest. Lunge your right leg forward, bending both knees.

b. Rotate your head, neck, shoulders, and torso to the right, keeping the weight at chest level while leaning your torso forward slightly. Push off your right foot and step back to the starting position. Repeat, lunging forward with your left leg and turning your upper body to the left. Do 10 to 12 reps per side.

FORM TIP! Keep your front knee over your ankle and your shoulders squared above your hips as you lunge.

Make it easier: If you're having difficulty keeping your balance, just do the alternating lunge without the rotation.

④ Chest Press/Fly Combo

(works: chest)

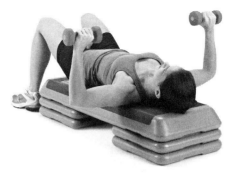

a. Lie faceup on a step or bench. (Option: If you don't have a bench, lie on the floor and position a large pillow or sofa cushion vertically under your back.) Hold medium or light weights with your arms extended above your chest, palms forward. Slowly bend your elbows, lowering your arms out to the sides until your elbows are at chest level. Straighten your arms again.

b. Rotate your arms so your palms face each other. Slowly lower your arms out to the sides to chest level, elbows slightly bent. Lift the weights above your chest again. Repeat the press/fly combo for a total of 10 to 12 reps.

FORM TIP! During the fly (b) part of the move, move the weights in an arc that is in line with your chest; don't bring them too far forward or back.

⑤ Squat with Triceps Kickback

(works: quads, glutes, triceps)

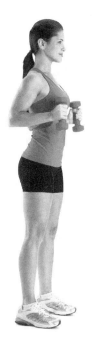

a. Stand with your feet hip-distance apart, holding light weights next to your chest with your elbows bent behind you.

b. Push your butt back, bending your knees about 90 degrees (or as far as you can) as if sitting in a chair (you should be able to see your toes if you look down). As you lower down, press the weights behind you, keeping your arms close to your body. Stand up and return to the starting position, bringing your hands back toward your chest. Repeat the squat/kickback combo, doing 12 to 15 reps.

FORM TIP! Try not to arch your neck—keep your head in line with your spine—and keep your body weight over your heels. Start with your arms bent so that when you squat down, you straighten your arms and work your legs and arms at the same time.

6 Curtsy Lunge with Lateral Raise

(works: shoulders, quads, glutes)

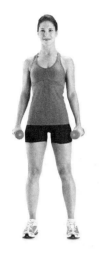

a. Stand with your feet hip-distance apart, holding light weights with your arms at your sides, your palms facing your body. Cross your right leg behind you, as if in a curtsy, bending your left knee 90 degrees. Keep your left knee over your ankle.

b. As you bend your knees, lift your arms out to the sides to shoulder height, keeping your elbows slightly bent. Straighten your legs and lower your arms as you return to the starting position. Do 10 to 12 reps, switch legs, and repeat.

FORM TIP! Keep your knee aligned over your ankle and your shin vertical to the floor. Keep your torso upright and hips and shoulders as square as possible.

Make it easier:
Do the lunges and lateral lifts separately.

Plié Squat with Heel Lift and Biceps Curl

(works: outer thighs, quads, glutes, calves, biceps)

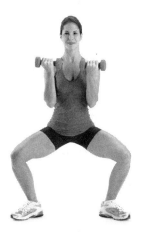

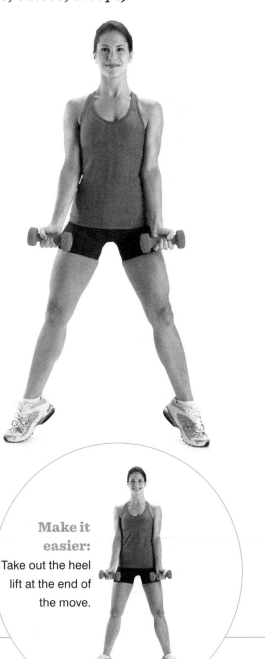

a. Stand with your feet just wider than shoulder-distance apart, toes turned out, holding light or medium weights in front of your thighs with your palms away from your body. Bend your knees 90 degrees, keeping them in the same direction as your toes, with your chest tall and abs tight. As you bend your knees, curl the weights toward your shoulders. Stand up and lower the weights.

b. Rise up onto the balls of your feet for one count, keeping the weights in front of your thighs. Lower your heels and repeat the plié/lift /curl combo. Do 12 to 15 reps.

FORM TIP! Don't allow your knees to collapse in as you bend your legs; try pressing your knees out to the sides.

Make it easier: Take out the heel lift at the end of the move.

8 Bridge/Hamstring Curl

(works: hamstrings, glutes)

a. Lie faceup on the floor, knees bent with your heels on the floor, arms at your sides with your palms facing down. Place a paper plate or sheet of paper under your left foot. Engage your abs to stabilize your core and lift your hips, being careful not to arch your back. Hold for one count, then lower to the starting position and repeat. Do 12 to 15 reps.

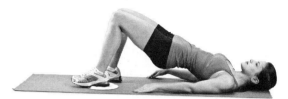

b. On your final rep, keep your hips lifted. Slowly slide your left foot forward, keeping your hips steady and right foot in place, then slide your left foot back toward your body. Do 10 to 12 reps, then switch legs and repeat.

FORM TIP! If you have a stability ball, you can also do the bridge move with your feet on the ball and your legs straight, then use your heels to bring the ball toward your butt for the curl (see page 314).

Make it easier:
Just do the hip lift and take out the hamstring curl.

9 Plank Combo

(works: abs, obliques)

a. (not shown) Lie facedown on the floor, your elbows under your shoulders with your forearms on the floor, fingers facing forward, and legs extended behind you. With your feet about hip-distance apart, flex your ankles so your toes are on the floor and your heels face the ceiling (see photo on page 110). Lift your hips, forming a straight line from head to heels, keeping abs tight. Hold for 15 to 20 seconds.

b. Rotate to the right side, lifting your right arm above your right shoulder. Keep your left forearm on the floor and turn it to face forward. Keep your body aligned and your legs stacked. Hold for 15 to 20 seconds.

c. (not shown) Lower for one count and switch sides, lifting your hips and rotating to the left as you lift your left arm above your shoulder, body aligned, and balance on your right forearm and stacked legs. Hold for 15 to 20 seconds.

FORM TIP! Keep your hips lifted and abs engaged throughout the exercise.

Make it easier: Do the front plank (a) from a full pushup position, your arms straight. For the side plank (b and c), cross your top leg over your bottom one so both feet are on the floor.

10 Crunch Series

(works: abdominals, obliques)

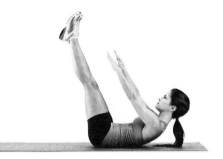

a. Lie faceup on the floor, arms at your sides. Lift your legs above your hips. Holding your legs here, lift your head, neck, and shoulders off the floor, reaching your hands toward your feet. Do 15 to 20 reps.

b. Lower your upper body for one count, then reach your hands toward the outside of your left leg. Do 15 to 20 reps, then repeat, reaching toward the outside of your right leg.

FORM TIP! Keep a space the size of a tennis ball between your chin and chest; make the movement come from your trunk, not your neck.

Make it easier:
Bend your knees.

FAT-BURNING CARDIO INTERVALS

Week 2

This week we'll build on the intervals you did last week, making the intensity bursts a little longer while keeping the recovery time steady. Your work time is now just as long as your rest time. Try to make your work intervals just a little harder this week, bumping up your RPE by 1 point. On your heart rate monitor, aim for 10 to 15 beats higher than your VT1 during the intervals. This will help challenge you to work at a higher level, improving both your overall fitness and your VT1, while still giving you enough time to recover.

Remember, you don't want to work so hard that you're barely able to speak. During the work intervals, you should be able to quickly count to 15 (about 4 seconds) out loud without pausing to take a breath. Do this workout at least twice this week, adding an optional third session if you have time.

MINUTES	INTENSITY	TALK TEST	HEART RATE (OPTIONAL)	RPE
0–3	Light (warmup)	Easy conversation	Below VT1	3–4
3–7	Medium-high	Challenging (short phrases)	10–15 beats above VT1	7–8
7–11	Medium	Easier (short sentences)	Just below VT1	5
11–15	Medium-high	Challenging (short phrases)	10–15 beats above VT1	7–8
15–19	Medium	Easier (short sentences)	Just below VT1	5
19–23	Medium-high	Challenging (short phrases)	10–15 beats above VT1	7–8
23–27	Medium	Easier (short sentences)	Just below VT1	5
27–30	Light (cooldown)	Easy (full conversation)	Below VT1	3–4

More Ways to Fight Fat

Diet and regular exercise aren't the only ways to help reduce body fat. Try incorporating some of these healthy habits to slim down and shed pounds.

TAKE A COMMERCIAL BREAK. An Australian study found that people who took the greatest number of breaks during otherwise sedentary behavior (like watching TV) had a 16 percent lower waist circumference than those who made a more permanent indentation on the couch cushions, regardless of whether they had a regular workout routine. Even just walking around for a minute or two was enough to make a difference.[2] It's not just for your waistline: Other studies have shown that too much sitting can create some unhealthy physiological changes that can lead to obesity, diabetes, heart disease, and a higher rate of mortality.[3]

GET A GOOD NIGHT'S SLEEP. There's ample evidence that being well rested can make for a slimmer silhouette. Several studies have shown that when you cut back on pillow time, you're more likely to have a higher BMI. One recent study from the University of Chicago Medical Center found that when dieters got a full night's sleep, about half of the weight they lost came from fat. When they cut back on sleep, only one-fourth of the weight loss came from fat.[4] Researchers speculate that when we don't get enough sleep, we produce more of the hunger hormone ghrelin—so even if you're more active during the day, you may be more likely to grab a big bag of chips than a handful of carrots.

STAY CONNECTED. Instead of reaching for a snack, pick up the phone the next time you're feeling hungry. Research on female monkeys shows that social stress and isolation may lead to higher levels of central fat deposits, as well as higher levels of the stress hormones linked to belly fat.[5]

CHEW SOME SUGAR-FREE GUM. It'll help more than just your breath. Researchers from the University of Rhode Island found that subjects who chewed gum for a total of 1 hour in the morning (broken into three 20-minute chewing sessions) consumed 67 fewer calories at lunch and didn't make up for it by eating more later in the day. They also expended about 5 percent more energy and felt more energized after chewing gum.[6]

WALK WHENEVER POSSIBLE. The more steps you take, the more calories you burn—and that doesn't mean spending all your time on the treadmill. Try to work in more walking throughout your day. Visit a coworker in person instead of sending an e-mail; take the stairs an extra couple of flights; park your car as far from an entrance as possible. Just six 5-minute walks a day can add up to about 100 calories, which can make a difference of about 10 pounds a year.

LISA MILLER

Age: 64

Height: 5'4"

Pounds lost: 8½

Inches lost: 5½

What she's most proud of: "I've gotten into some healthy habits for good—I want to exercise every day!"

Favorite foods: Quinoa with mint and lemon; air-popped popcorn with Old Bay Seasoning

Lisa Miller never really had a weight problem until she moved from New York City—where her feet were her main method of transportation—to Pennsylvania. "I went from walking everywhere and being highly active to driving in my car all the time," she says.

A health scare (she had surgery to remove two benign brain tumors in mid-2009, followed by an aneurism 2 months later) didn't help matters, as she was forced to stay inside and recover for several months. Lisa gained about 20 pounds in a year. "I started to eat everything and anything because I figured if I was going to die, at least I'd enjoy myself with a doughnut." Soon she topped 188 pounds.

When the doctors gave her the all-

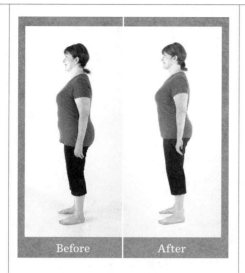

Before | After

clear to start moving again, Lisa got back into exercise big time, joining a local walking club, swimming, and doing water aerobics at least three times a week. But the weight, which had come on so easily, just wasn't coming off.

"I've always done either a diet or an exercise program but never tried to do both together," she says. On the Turn Up Your Fat Burn plan, she found having to watch her portion size and do both strength and cardio made a big difference.

Doing circuit training gave her a new perspective on building strength. "I loved that you keep moving the whole time. When I lifted weights in the past, I always got kind of lazy by the second or third set. But when you do the moves in a cycle, it's like you're starting fresh with each set, so I worked harder each time through." She also saw a big improvement in her balance and upper-body strength. Lisa did the cardio intervals ("I'm jogging for the first time since I got sick 2 years ago," she reports) and also kept up with her water aerobics and Pilates classes.

In 1 month, Lisa dropped 8½ pounds and lost 2 inches off her waist, 1½ inches off her hips, and another 1¼ inches off her thighs. "I'm no longer wearing big, over-size shirts that hide my shape—all my clothes fit me better now," says Lisa. "I'm wearing pants I couldn't get into in over a year and can't wait to put on a new gym outfit I just bought. And all the ladies in my aqua aerobic class say I look better in my swimsuit."

Tracking her foods and eating small, regular meals along with snacks helped Lisa get a handle on her appetite. "Now I never miss a snack—I carry something small with me, like some almonds or cereal, so I don't get too hungry later in the day." Having a sense of portion size was also important: "I finally got a sense of how much I should be eating at one time." She also swapped green tea for diet soda and says it's her new favorite drink.

"The good habits I've started are sticking with me—I'm eating better, keeping up with the strength and cardio, and getting a handle on my appetite. I want to keep my goals modest and doable so they're not only achievable but actually last!"

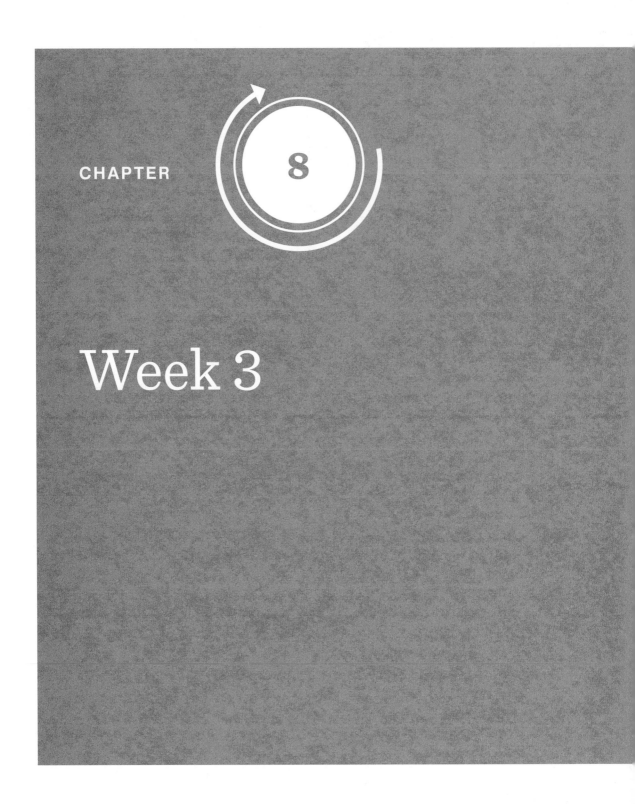

CHAPTER

8

Week 3

It's Week 3, which means you're halfway through the 4-week program! We're continuing to build on the efforts made during the prior 2 weeks, adding more intensity to the strength workouts and making the cardio intervals a little more challenging. Keep up the good work!

YOUR GOALS THIS WEEK

- Do two metabolic strength circuit workouts (two or three times through; about 35 to 45 minutes per session).
- Do two fat-burning cardio interval workouts (about 30 minutes each).
- **Optional:** Do one fat-burning cardio interval workout (about 30 minutes).

Here's what a sample week looks like.

Monday: Metabolic strength circuit

Tuesday: Cardio intervals

Wednesday: Off

Thursday: Metabolic strength circuit plus optional cardio intervals

Friday: Off

Saturday: Cardio intervals

Sunday: Optional additional activity (golf, hiking, cycling, etc.)

Begin with your warmup and stretch series. Then do the exercises in the order given, resting about 15 seconds between moves and a full 90 seconds at the end of the circuit. Complete the circuit at least two times through, doing an optional third circuit if time allows.

WARMUP AND STRETCH

March or jog in place or go for a walk at a comfortable pace for 3 to 5 minutes. You should be able to maintain an easy conversation, but go fast enough that it doesn't feel like you're window shopping.

Then do the dynamic stretches starting on page 61 for about 30 seconds each, moving at your own pace. Keep the movements under control.

After the workout: Finish by doing the static stretches on page 75.

METABOLIC STRENGTH CIRCUIT

Week 3

Now that you're halfway through the program and have done the strength circuits several times, we're going to increase the challenge again by adding on some balance exercises and plyometric (jumping) moves to build core strength and

Get a Jump Start!

Jumping looks simple, but it can be hard on your joints if you're not careful. Stay safe with these tips on how to leap lightly.

○ Land softly. Try to land on the middle of your foot, then let your weight fall back on your heels. The midfoot is better equipped to handle the impact than the ball of your foot or the heel.

○ As you land, try to push your hips back and down, which will allow some of your bigger muscles to absorb more of the impact.

○ Don't lock your knees when you land; they should always be at least slightly bent.

○ Try to keep your knees aligned over your second toe—for women especially, this will help reduce the injury risk that can come with having a wider Q angle (the angle at which the upper leg meets the lower leg).

○ Keep your abs tight to protect your spine, and land with your trunk slightly forward and your head in line with your spine or looking upward slightly.

increase your calorie burn. If you can, you may also want to choose slightly heavier weights than you used the past 2 weeks. If you don't have heavier weights at home, add a couple of reps to what you did last week.

Remember to progress at your own pace. If a move feels too difficult or challenging to complete with the proper form, substitute a similar move from Week 1 or 2 (or just repeat either of those week's full circuits). Do this workout two times this week on nonconsecutive days.

What you'll need: Light and medium weights, a sturdy chair or bench, and a mat (optional).

1 Lunge, Turn, and Lift

(works: quads, glutes, hamstrings, obliques)

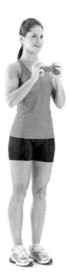

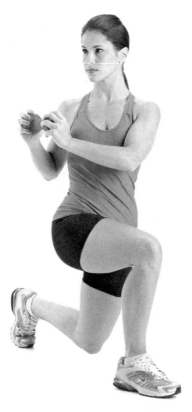

a. Stand tall, holding a medium weight in front of your chest with both hands. Lunge your right leg forward, bending both knees (keep your right knee above your right ankle and your shoulders above your hips).

b. Rotate your arms, head, neck, shoulders, and torso to the right.

c. Step your left foot forward, lifting your left knee to hip height. Balance on your right leg for one count. Lunge forward with your left leg; repeat the series. Do 12 to 15 reps per side.

FORM TIP! Not a lot of room to move around? After you do the lunge/lift leading with your right leg, turn around and do the same move, this time stepping forward with your left leg.

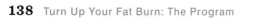

Make it easier:
If balancing is difficult, bring your feet together and then lift your leg.

Jumping Squat

(works: glutes, quads, core)

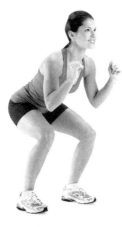

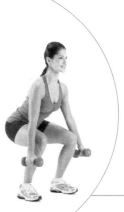

a. Stand with your feet hip-distance apart, your arms at your sides (no weights). Squat down, bending your knees about 90 degrees and keeping your weight over your heels (you should be able to see your toes if you look down).

b. Jump up, swinging your arms above your head, and land in a squat with your knees bent. Immediately jump again, landing in a squat. Do 15 to 20 reps.

FORM TIP! Land softly with your knees bent; move into the next squat as quickly as possible.

Make it easier:
If jumping doesn't feel good, do the dumbbell squat in Week 1, using slightly heavier weights.

③ Single-Leg Deadlift with Touchdown

(works: hamstrings, glutes, shoulders)

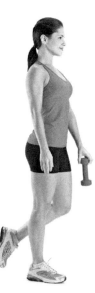

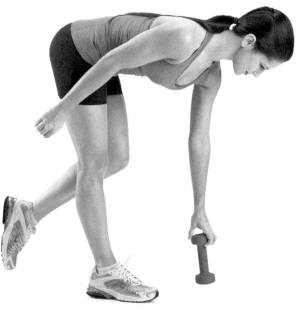

a. Stand with your feet together, your left hand holding a medium weight to your left side. Balance on your right foot, keeping your knee slightly bent.

b. Hinge forward from the waist, keeping your right knee slightly bent. Touch the dumbbell to the floor, bracing your abdominals; keep your torso parallel with the floor and your hips level. (You'll feel the movement along the back of your right leg.) Pull back up to start and repeat. Do 10 to 12 reps; switch sides and repeat.

FORM TIP! Keep your abs firm and your back straight to help with balance. Don't allow your torso to rotate.

Make it easier:
If balancing here is difficult, do a regular Romanian deadlift with both feet on the floor as in Week 1, using slightly heavier weights.

④ Balancing Alternating Biceps Curl

(works: biceps, core, glutes)

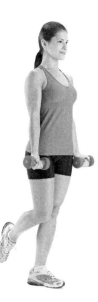

a. Stand tall with your arms at your sides, palms facing out and holding light or medium weights. Balance on your left foot.

b. Curl your right hand toward your right shoulder, then lower it as you curl your left hand toward your left shoulder. Continue, alternating arms, for a total of 8 to 10 reps per side. Then switch legs, balancing on your right foot. Repeat curls for another 8 to 10 reps per side.

FORM TIP! Help your balance by concentrating on a spot on the floor a few feet in front of you. Remember to switch legs halfway through the set.

Make it easier: Keep both feet on the floor (or touch your foot down to the floor as needed).

⑤ Balancing Shoulder Press/Triceps Extension

(works: shoulders, triceps, core, glutes)

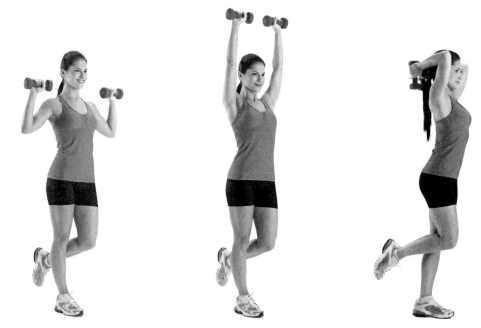

a. Stand with your feet together, holding light or medium weights at shoulder height, palms facing forward with your elbows in the 4 and 8 o'clock positions. Balance on your right foot, keeping the knee slightly bent.

b. Press the weights up, keeping your abs tight. Lower and repeat. Do 12 to 15 reps.

c. Switch legs, balancing on your left foot. Rotate your arms so that your palms face each other, keeping your weights close together above your head. Bend your elbows and lower the weights behind your head, keeping your arms close to your ears. Straighten and repeat. Do 12 to 15 reps. Then switch legs again and repeat the press/extension on the opposite sides.

FORM TIP! Keeping your abs pulled in can help you maintain balance. Remember to switch legs between the shoulder press and triceps extension.

Make it easier: Keep both feet on the floor (or touch your foot down to the floor as needed).

⑥ Scissor Lunge
(works: quads, glutes, calves)

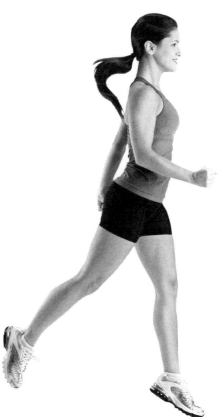

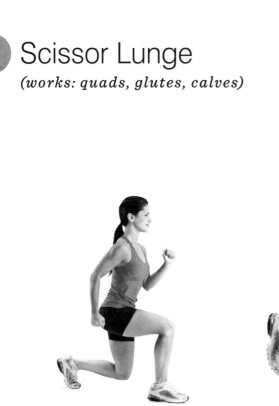

a. Stand with your feet hip-distance apart, your arms at your sides (no weights). Take a short step (no more than 24 inches) forward with your right foot as if lunging, hinging your hips and lowering yourself toward the floor until your knees are bent about 90 degrees.

b. Explode up, switching legs in the air so you land with your left foot lunged forward. Immediately repeat, switching legs so your right foot is forward. Do 10 reps per leg.

FORM TIP! Don't lean too far forward when you jump, and land in a lunge position with your knees bent and your front knee over the ankle; use your arms for momentum.

Make it easier:
If jumping is uncomfortable or too difficult, do regular stationary lunges as in Week 1, using slightly heavier weights.

7 Standing Halo

(works: core stabilizers, shoulders)

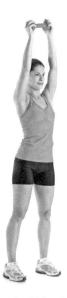

Stand with your feet hip-distance apart, holding one medium weight horizontally with your arms extended above your head, elbows bent. Slowly draw a big circle above your head with both hands, moving in a clockwise direction. Make 10 circles, then reverse directions.

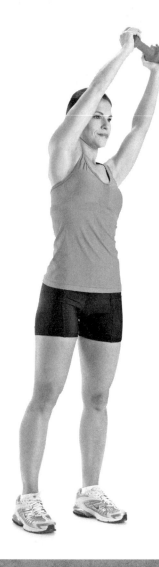

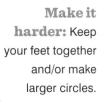

Make it harder: Keep your feet together and/or make larger circles.

FORM TIP! Try to keep your torso and lower body still as you move your arms and shoulders.

8 Reverse Lunge with Double-Arm Row

(works: quads, glutes, calves, upper back)

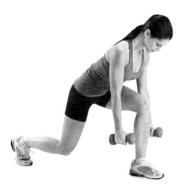

a. (not shown) Stand with your feet hip-distance apart, your arms at your sides, holding medium weights. Lunge back with your right foot, bending both knees 90 degrees; keep your left knee above your left ankle.

b. Lean forward from your waist, keeping your back flat and abs engaged as you bring your chest toward your knees.

c. Draw both elbows past your ribs, keeping your arms close to your sides. Straighten your arms, then stand up, pushing off the left foot to step back to start. Do 10 reps of the lunge/row combo; switch sides and repeat.

FORM TIP! Keep your back flat and abs engaged as you lean forward from the waist to do the row.

Make it easier: If doing the lunge/row together seems too difficult, do the lunges with one side first, then hold on the final rep and do the rows; switch legs and repeat.

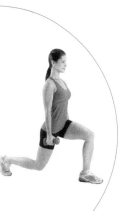

⑨ Step Up with Lateral Raise

(works: quads, glutes, outer thighs, shoulders)

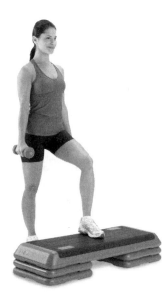

a. Stand in front of a step, bench, or sturdy low chair, holding light weights at your sides. Place your left foot on the step or bench.

b. Step up with your right foot, bringing your arms out to the sides at shoulder height, elbows slightly bent. Step your right foot back to start while lowering your arms, then step down with the left foot. Repeat with opposite legs. Do 10 to 15 reps, alternating legs.

FORM TIP! Keep your elbows slightly bent as you raise your arms out to the sides, and engage your abs as you step up and down.

Make it harder:
Add a balance challenge by lifting your back foot to hip height as you step up onto the bench.

10 Standing Torso Twist

(works: obliques)

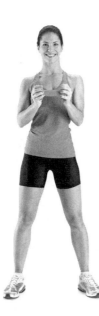

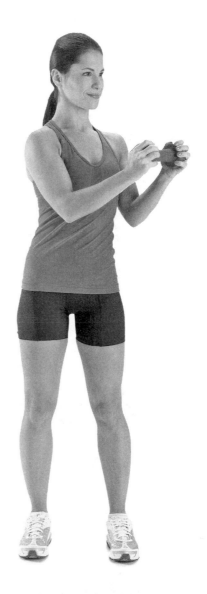

a. Stand with your feet 6 to 12 inches apart, your hands in front of your chest, and hold a medium weight horizontally with both hands.

b. Rotate your upper body and head to the left as far as possible, holding for a moment without bouncing, then rotate back to center. Repeat, rotating to the right and back to center. Continue rotating left and right; do 15 to 20 rotations per side.

FORM TIP! Keep your lower body still and your hips facing forward throughout the exercise; the movement should come from your core.

⑪ Side Lunge with Kick

(works: quads, glutes, hamstrings, outer thighs, core)

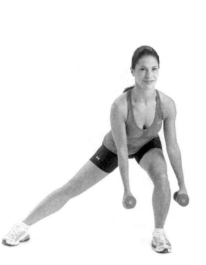

a. Stand with your feet hip-distance apart, arms at your sides, holding light or medium weights. Step your left foot about 24 inches to the left side, keeping your weight over your heels and both feet facing forward. Shift your hips back as you bend your left knee 90 degrees. (Your right leg stays straight; most of your body weight is shifted into your left hip.) Lower the weights toward your left ankle.

b. Step the right foot forward to meet the left, and then kick your right leg powerfully to the side as you lean to the left; bring the weights toward your chest to help counterbalance. Lower your right leg and repeat. Do 10 lunge/kick combos; switch sides.

FORM TIP! During the side lunge, make sure your left knee is aligned between the second and third toes of your left foot and the shin is perpendicular to the floor. You should feel the movement along the left side of your butt. During the kick, you'll feel it along the right side of your butt.

Make it easier: Take out the kick and just step feet together.

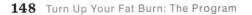

FAT-BURNING CARDIO INTERVALS

Week 3

Now that you're halfway through the program, it's time to increase the intensity of your cardio. This week, the "work" half of the interval is 5 minutes long, while recovery time is 4 minutes (1.25:1 ratio). Increasing interval length will help push your VT1, so you can burn more fat at a higher effort level (and ultimately burn more calories).

Your RPE during the work part of the interval should feel like 7 or 8 on a scale of 1 to 10—hard enough that your breathing is choppy but not so hard that you can't speak at all. Aim to keep your heart rate about 10 to 15 beats above VT1. Do this workout at least twice this week, with an optional third session.

MINUTES	INTENSITY	TALK TEST	HEART RATE (OPTIONAL)	RPE
0–3	Light (warmup)	Easy conversation	Below VT1	3–4
3–8	Medium-high	Challenging (short phrases)	10–15 beats above VT1	8
8–12	Medium	Easier (short sentences)	Just below VT1	5
12–17	Medium-high	Challenging (short phrases)	10–15 beats above VT1	8
17–21	Medium	Easier (short sentences)	Just below VT1	5
21–26	Medium-high	Challenging (short phrases)	10–15 beats above VT1	8
26–32	Medium	Easier (short sentences)	Just below VT1	5
32–34	Light (cooldown)	Easy (full conversation)	Below VT1	3–4

Conquer Your Cravings

The best weight-loss intentions aren't always a match for a powerful craving. Sometimes the lure of the candy bowl can be too much to resist, especially when you're trying to cut back on calories. And if you're stressed-out about work or family or are out celebrating a special occasion, even the strongest willpower can weaken. No surprise that for many women, the top draws are chocolate, salty snacks, chips, and french fries, according to a study from Tufts University in Boston.[7] Here's how to stay strong.

Don't make your diet too restrictive. The Turn Up Your Fat Burn diet is designed to give you an adequate amount of both fat and carbohydrates. Both of these are important to keep you from straying too far down the deep-fried path. Some healthy fats (like nuts and avocados) can keep you feeling satisfied longer. Also, having enough carbs (fruits, veggies, whole grains) will bathe your brain in feel-good serotonin so you won't reach for the cookie jar.

Watch for emotional eating. No surprise: We tend to eat more (and more out of control) when we're under stress. Often we're not even aware of how many calories we're consuming. Keeping a food log can help you track your eating behavior—take note of your hunger level, what you ate, and how you felt before and afterward. Reviewing the log can help you pinpoint whether you're eating because of emotion (angry, sad, stressed-out) or true hunger.

Reward yourself. Treat yourself to a manicure, download a new song, take some time to talk to a friend, or get lost in a new novel. When you start to associate other behaviors with pleasure, you'll take away some of the power of the foods you crave.

Plan in advance. A party or sporting event can melt the resolve of even the most iron-willed dieter. Bring along some fresh fruit or a healthy snack, and plan to drink a nonalcoholic beverage, like seltzer with lime or a splash of OJ. Work out a strategy in advance so you will be prepared for a dietary distraction when it comes.

Go ahead, have a little. Don't entirely avoid the foods you crave. If you really want chocolate, have a single-serving piece so you can savor the flavor (splurge for really good chocolate; it's worth it). Indulging a little now and then will keep you from going overboard later. The exception: If you're craving a food that you know to be a trigger food—one that will set you off on an eating frenzy—stay away. Substitute a similar treat (in a single-serving size) so you don't have any extras around to tease you later.

Say *om*. Researchers at the Fred Hutchinson Cancer Center in Seattle found that people who practice yoga are more mindful about what they eat and less likely to give in to cravings.[8] Yoga seems to make you more aware of your body, as well as more in tune with what you eat and why. You don't have to sign on with an ashram; in the study, a half hour of yoga practice a week was enough to make a difference.

KIMBERLY HAMPSEY

Age: 43

Height: 5′7″

Pounds lost: $7\frac{1}{2}$

Inches lost: $2\frac{3}{4}$

What she's most proud of:
"I was getting sluggish and didn't care what I looked like. Now I feel like I've had a tune-up and I'm back on track!"

Favorite new foods: Low-fat Greek yogurt with fresh blueberries; flat-bread pizza with grilled chicken

When Kimberly (Kim) and her husband decided to relocate from Texas to their native Pennsylvania, they knew it might be a little stressful. They just didn't anticipate quite how much upheaval it was going to cause: "It took over a year to sell our place in Houston, so we were paying two mortgages." To cope, Kim snacked on whatever she could find. "I didn't care what I ate and barely worked out—I thought we were going to move, so I quit my gym membership."

When they did finally make the move up north, Kim celebrated by enjoying all her local childhood favorites: pierogies, cheesesteaks, and shoofly pie. "I work

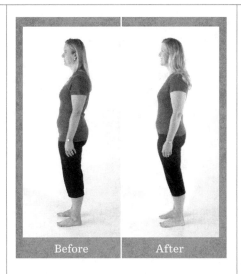

Before   After

out of my home, so all these foods were always around me," says Kim, who soon hit 172 pounds. "I definitely needed to make a change!"

Kim liked having a structured program to get her back into a regular routine—but she didn't want to take hours away from her busy workday. She carefully planned her workouts. "Knowing that I could get to the gym, do the workout, and be back at my desk in less than an hour was huge," she says. "And I'd always feel so much better when I was done."

One key motivator for Kim: keeping a food log. "When I'm tired or bored or don't want to start a new work project, the kitchen is always right there. Having to write everything down put it in black and white for me, and soon I started noticing patterns, like when I ate more out of boredom than hunger."

After a couple of weeks on the plan, Kim noticed she could jog and even run the cardio intervals more easily. Doing the resistance workouts improved her core strength enough to make a difference in her golf game and relieved her back pain.

She kept up the routine even when her work took her on the road. "I bought some healthy snacks at a store near my hotel, and I was able to do all the workouts in the hotel gym."

After 4 weeks, Kim had already dropped one clothing size (and in some cases two!). The workouts also improved her muscle tone. "I love that the backs of my arms don't look droopy."

Having a set routine also helped Kim through a rough stretch coping with two sudden deaths in the family. "Exercising was a huge stress reliever," she recalls. "It was an hour or so I could just focus on myself."

About 3 months after starting the plan, Kim had lost a full 20 pounds and ran her first 5-K race in less than 36 minutes. She thinks she'll even get back into swimming. "From age 5 to 21, I swam competitively. Then I got to the point that I couldn't even imagine putting on a bathing suit. Now I think I'm ready to walk around in one again!"

Week 4

You've made it to the 4th week of the program—congratulations! It may be the final week in this plan, but don't consider it as your final week of fitness. Think of this as simply the end of your first step toward a lifetime of better health and the beginning of a new journey of continued self-discovery.

By now we hope you've come to enjoy the experience and have started to notice some very real and lasting changes in your body and in your fitness and energy levels. After doing 3 full weeks of the plan, don't be afraid to take the intensity up another notch. It's rewarding to be able to challenge yourself and see what you're capable of. (Don't sell yourself short—you can do a lot more than you may think you can!) That said, please modify the plan as appropriate to make sure it works for you.

YOUR GOALS THIS WEEK

○ Do two metabolic strength circuit workouts (two or three times through, about 40 to 60 minutes per session).

○ Do two fat-burning cardio interval workouts (about 35 minutes each).

○ **Optional:** Do one optional fat-burning cardio interval workout (about 35 minutes).

Here's what a sample week looks like.

Monday: Metabolic strength circuit

Tuesday: Off

Wednesday: Cardio intervals

Thursday: Off

Friday: Metabolic strength circuit plus optional cardio intervals

Saturday: Optional additional activity (golf, hiking, cycling, etc.)

Sunday: Cardio Intervals

DYNAMIC WARMUP

This week we're departing from the usual warmup for a higher-energy routine. Do these exercises just once at the beginning of each workout this week, then immediately move on to the metabolic strength circuit on page 160.

After the workout: Finish with the static stretches on page 75.

1 Cat Back/Down Dog

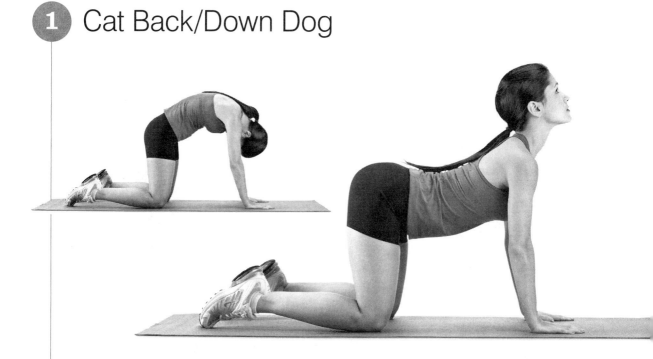

a. Begin on your hands and knees. Exhaling slowly, round your back, contracting your abdominals and tucking your pelvis under. Hold for a moment.

b. Relax, then slowly inhale and reverse the movement, arching your back, lifting your tailbone up and your chest forward while raising your head. Hold for a moment.

c. (not shown) Return to the starting position on your hands and knees, with your spine neutral.

d. Lift your hips toward the ceiling, extending your arms and legs while pressing your heels toward the floor. Allow your head to drop between your arms. Hold for a moment; drop your legs and return to all fours. Repeat the entire series 5 to 10 times.

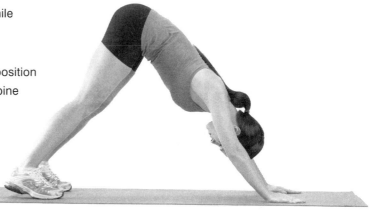

② Bodyweight Squat and Arm Reach

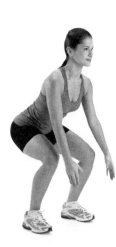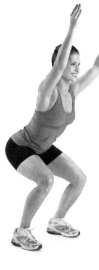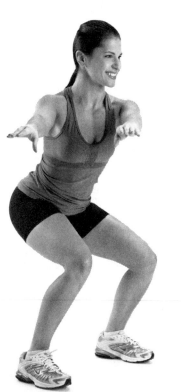

a. Stand with your feet hip-distance apart, your arms at your sides (no weights). Squat down, bending your knees about 90 degrees or as deeply as you can, reaching your hands toward the floor.

b. Repeat, this time reaching your arms overhead.

c. On the next rep, reach both hands toward the left side.

d. On the next rep, reach both hands to the right side. Repeat the entire squat series (down, up, side to side), switching directions for the reaches with each rep, for a total of 10 series.

③ Around-the-Clock Lunges

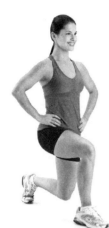
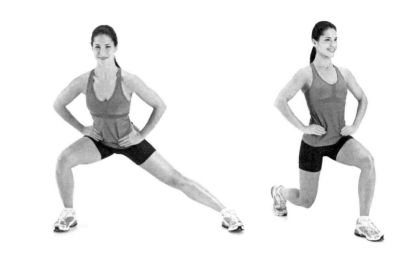

a. Stand as if you're in the center of a big clock. Lunge your right foot forward (12 o'clock), then step back to center.

b. Lunge your right foot to the side (3 o'clock), then step back to center.

c. Lunge your right foot back (6 o'clock), then step back to center.

d. Lunge your right foot crossed behind you in a curtsy lunge (7 o'clock), then step back to center. Switch legs after you complete the series; do the series on each leg 5 times.

METABOLIC STRENGTH CIRCUIT

Week 4

This week you'll step up the intensity of your strength routine by working the muscles in different ways while also cutting back on your recovery time between each move. We're doing compound sets here, which means two exercises per muscle group. For the first exercise, you'll move primarily in a linear (up and down) movement; in the second, you'll add some rotation to work the muscles in a different way (and also bring other muscle groups in on the action).

Because the movements and exercises will be a bit more challenging, it's even more important to get your body ready for action. That's why we introduced the dynamic warmup moves you've just learned, which are designed to get you ready for the work ahead by boosting your heart rate and bringing your joints and muscles through a full range of motion. Do them just once.

After you do the dynamic stretches on pages 157–159, do the metabolic strength circuit two times through, this time resting for just 10 seconds between each move. Recover for a full minute between each circuit. If you have the time and energy, do a third circuit. Do this workout two times this week on nonconsecutive days.

What you'll need: Light and medium weights, a sturdy chair or bench, and a mat (optional).

① Burpee (Pushup/Squat/Jump Combo)

(works: arms, chest, core, quads, glutes)

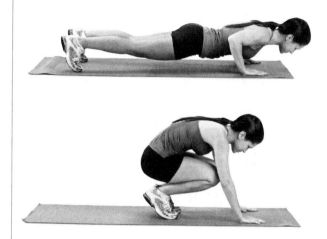
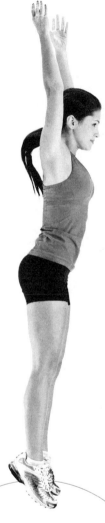

a. Begin in a full pushup position, your hands on the floor under your shoulders and your legs extended behind you, abs tight. Lower your chest toward the floor and push back to the starting position.

b. Jump both feet toward your hands.

c. Jump up, landing in a squat. Stand up and squat back down, then place your hands on the floor and jump your feet back to a pushup position. Do 5 push-up/jump/squat combos.

FORM TIP! Move through the exercise as quickly as possible, going from the pushup straight to the jump and squat. Land in the squat with your knees bent.

Make it easier:
If you have difficulty jumping, walk your feet back toward your hands, stand up and do a regular squat, then place your hands on the floor and walk your feet back until you're in a full pushup position. You can also do this as a modified pushup with your knees on the floor.

Decline Pushup

(works: chest, core)

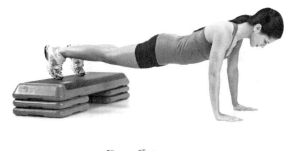

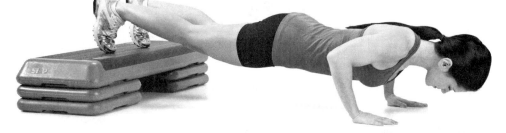

a. Place your feet on a bench or sturdy chair and your hands on the floor in a pushup position, shoulder-distance apart.

b. Bend your elbows, lowering your head toward the floor. Straighten and repeat. Do 8 to 10 reps.

FORM TIP! Keep your abs pulled in throughout the pushup to help maintain form.

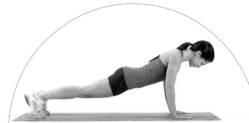

Make it easier:
If the decline movement is challenging, do a regular pushup with your feet on the floor or a modified pushup with your knees on the floor.

③ Standing Dumbbell Fly

(works: chest, core)

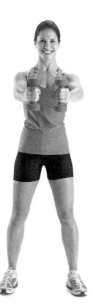

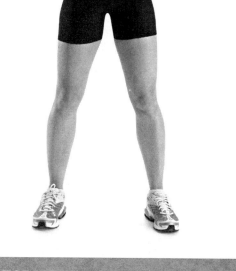

a. Stand holding medium weights with your arms in front at chest height, palms facing each other, and your elbows slightly bent.

b. Slowly bring the weights out to the sides, keeping them shoulder height, then return to the starting position. Do 10 to 12 reps.

FORM TIP! Keep the weights at chest height; try to keep your shoulders pressed down and back, not hunched up.

(4) Single-Leg Deadlift with Row

(works: hamstrings, glutes, upper back)

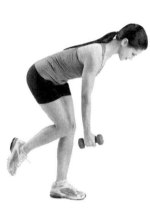

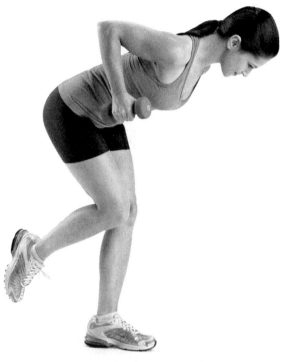

a. Stand with your feet together, holding a medium weight in your right hand at your side, your palm facing your body. Balance on your left foot, keeping your knee slightly bent. Hinge forward from your waist, keeping your left knee slightly bent and the weight directly under your right shoulder.

FORM TIP! Keep your arm close to your body and avoid rotating your torso; focus on a point on the floor to maintain balance.

b. Lift your right elbow toward your ribs, keeping your arm close to your body. Lower the weight, straightening your arm, then stand back up, staying balanced on your left foot. Repeat the deadlift/row combo 10 times; switch sides and repeat.

Make it easier:
If balancing is too challenging, do the exercise as a regular deadlift as in Week 1, adding in the row.

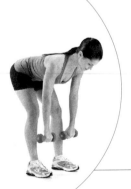

5 Reverse Lunge with Single-Arm High-Back Row

(works: quads, glutes, upper back)

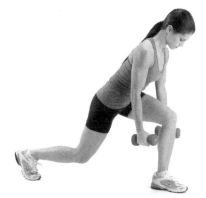

a. Stand holding medium weights with your feet hip-distance apart, your arms at your sides. Lunge back with your right foot, bending both knees 90 degrees; keep your left knee above your left ankle. Lean forward, extending both arms below your shoulders, your palms facing your body.

b. Lift just your right elbow past your ribs, keeping your arm close to your body (your left arm stays down). Lower your right arm and step back to the starting position. Do 10 reps of the lunge/row combo; switch sides and repeat.

FORM TIP! As you lunge back, keep your shoulders over your hips, then lean forward for the row. Keep your head in line with your spine and your back flat during the row.

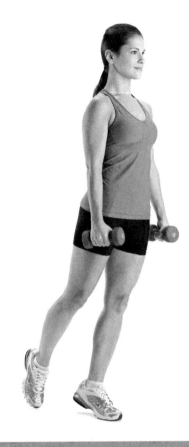

6 Single-Leg Squat with Heel Raise

(works: quads, glutes, calves)

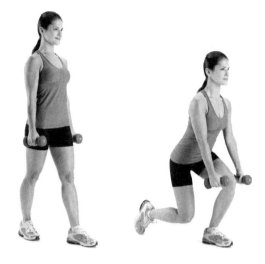

a. Stand holding medium weights with your palms facing your body and your feet staggered, your left foot forward as if taking a step.

b. Hinge forward slightly from the hips, pushing your butt backward, then lower your hips toward the floor, keeping most of your body weight on your left leg. (You should feel your left leg muscles working.) Continue lowering until your front thigh is parallel (or nearly) to the floor. Keep your left heel pressed into the floor and lift your right heel. Pause for a moment, then push upward, standing back up.

c. As you stand, rise up on the ball of your left foot; hold for 1 or 2 seconds, then lower and repeat. Do 12 to 15 reps; switch sides.

FORM TIP! Keep most of the weight on your front leg as you squat down, getting as low as you possibly can, or until your thigh is parallel to the floor.

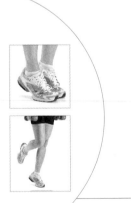

Make it easier:
If you find it too difficult to keep your balance here, do a regular squat, then raise both heels as you stand back up.

Make it harder:
Keep your back leg lifted throughout.

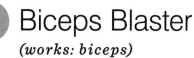

7 Biceps Blaster

(works: biceps)

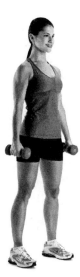

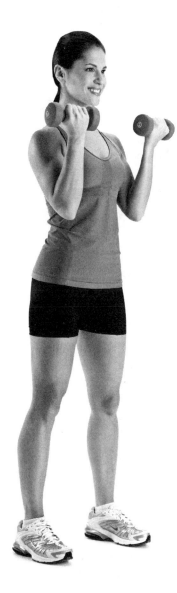

a. Stand holding weights with your arms at your sides, your palms facing your thighs.

b. Curl the weights toward your shoulders, rotating your arms as you lift the weights so your palms face your shoulders. Reverse the movement and repeat. Do 8 to 10 reps.

FORM TIP! Move slowly and evenly, taking two counts to lift the weights and two counts to lower them.

⑧ Concentration Biceps Curl

(works: biceps)

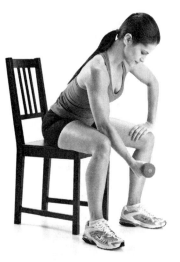

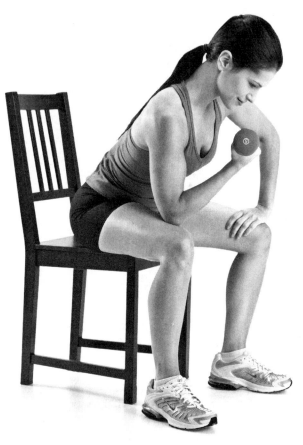

a. Sit on a sturdy chair or bench holding a medium weight in your right hand. Lean forward, placing your left hand on your left thigh and bringing your right elbow just inside your right thigh, your arm straight.

b. Curl the weight toward your shoulder. Hold for one count, then lower and repeat. Do 8 to 10 reps; switch sides and repeat.

Make it easier: Use a lighter weight than you did for the previous exercise.

FORM TIP! Use your inner thigh to brace your arm for the exercise. Move your arm through its full range of motion, pausing briefly at the top.

9 Advanced Triceps Dip

(works: triceps)

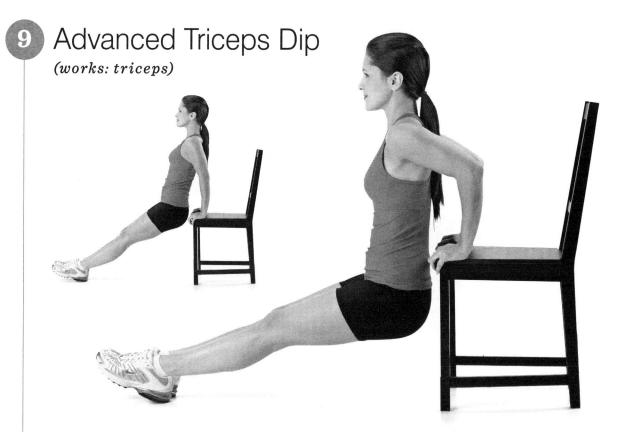

a. Sit on the edge of a sturdy chair or bench, your hands at the edge of the seat with your fingers facing forward. Straighten your legs, keeping your heels on the floor in front of you.

b. Lift your hips off the bench and lower your butt toward the floor, bending your elbows directly behind you. Straighten your arms and repeat the dip. Do 15 to 20 reps.

FORM TIP! Keep your hips and body close to the bench or chair as you lower yourself.

Make it easier:
Bend your knees 90 degrees (keeping your knees over your ankles) during the dip.

⑩ Overhead Triceps Extension

(works: triceps)

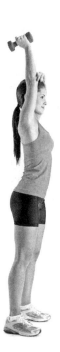

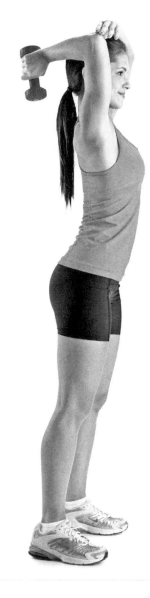

a. Stand holding a medium weight in your right hand, with your right arm extended and your left hand lightly touching your right elbow.

b. Bend your right elbow, bringing the weight behind your head. Straighten back to the starting position and repeat. Do 10 to 12 reps; switch sides and repeat.

FORM TIP! Use your opposite hand to provide support and keep the elbow of your working arm still during the exercise.

11 Wood Chop

(works: quads, glutes, obliques, shoulders)

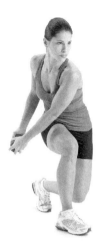

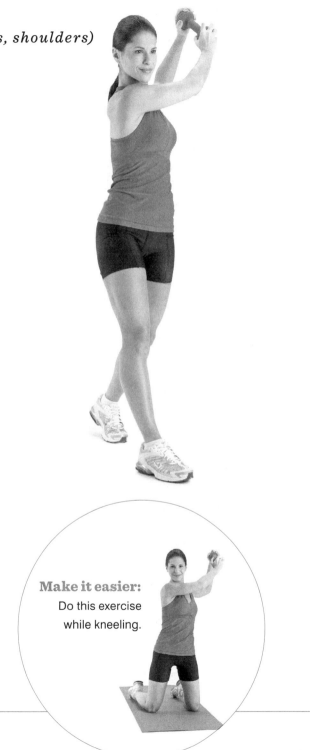

a. Stand holding a weight horizontally in front of you with both hands, with your right foot forward. Push your hips backward, then bend your knees into a squat. Rotate your hips and trunk to move the weight toward the outside of your right hip.

b. Press upward, rotating your hips and trunk while moving the weight diagonally across your body above your left shoulder. Repeat, lowering the dumbbell toward the outside of your right hip as you squat. Do 10 reps, then switch sides and repeat another 10 times.

FORM TIP! Move the weight diagonally from the floor toward the ceiling, with a full range of motion to work both your upper and lower body as well as your core.

Make it easier:
Do this exercise while kneeling.

12 Tabletop Twist

(works: obliques, glutes)

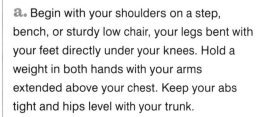

a. Begin with your shoulders on a step, bench, or sturdy low chair, your legs bent with your feet directly under your knees. Hold a weight in both hands with your arms extended above your chest. Keep your abs tight and hips level with your trunk.

b. Rotate your arms and torso to the left, lifting your right shoulder off the step until your arms are level with the floor. Pause for a moment, then rotate to the opposite side, keeping your hips elevated. Perform 15 to 20 reps per side.

> **FORM TIP!** Keep your hips lifted and squeeze your glutes to keep your lower back from sinking.

Stick-with-It Tips

Now that you're in the fourth week on the program, you may have already started to wonder . . . what's next? We have plenty of details and advice for you at the end of the book. For now, here's some advice on how to stay motivated for good.

Keep your support systems in place. Who or what has helped you stay on track for the past few weeks? Continue to enlist the aid of your friends and family: Make your workouts a group affair, have a healthy dinner party, take a lunchtime walk with a coworker.

If you get sidetracked, find your way back. We all have times when we veer off course. Don't let too many days off deter you. For your first couple of workouts, start gradually—half or two-thirds your previous level of effort—then increase the time or intensity with each new workout. Before long, you'll be back in the swing of it.

Set new goals. If your first goal was to complete this plan, then congrats— you're almost done! But make that goal the first of many. Weight loss experts recommend that the goals be "SMART." That's:

- **Specific:** Be as detailed as possible. "I will fit into my size 10 pants by September 1."
- **Measurable:** Set a goal you can monitor and evaluate.
- **Adjustable:** Have some flexibility to accommodate obstacles. Allow for potential setbacks and then get back into it.
- **Realistic**: If you're wearing a size 22 in July, it's not likely you're going to be in a 10 come September. Keep your goals grounded in reality—maybe plan on dropping just one size in 4 to 6 weeks.
- **Time-bound.** Give yourself a timeline for achieving this goal. How many workouts will you do this week? How long will it take to ultimately reach your goal?

Put it in black-and-white. Write down your goals and post them where you can see them. Clearly visualizing your goal can help you reach it. You can also post some positive affirmations around your house to remind you of your goals.

FAT-BURNING CARDIO INTERVALS

Week 4

This week's cardio is a little different from the previous 3 weeks, when you primarily worked at and just above VT1. With this workout, you'll push past VT1 toward VT2—an even higher intensity level at which you will really feel the burn. This is a bit more of a butt-kicking workout, which makes it a good way to work on your overall fitness and wake up your body.

These speed intervals last just 20 seconds, so make them count: You'll get another 40 seconds to recover (although you'll still work at a medium-high intensity) before starting again. There are seven very high-intensity bursts altogether. If you're on a treadmill or other cardio machine, jack up the speed or resistance to a fairly high level (rather than gradually increasing it). Try to challenge yourself: Since the intervals are short, you want to make sure you're working at as high of an intensity as you can for a brief period. You'll continue to work at and above VT1 for a good portion of the workout, so you'll be burning plenty of fat along the way.

You'll be doing this workout at least twice this week, with an optional third session.

Need for Speed

Make your intervals count! If you're doing the workout walking or jogging outside, speed up to a jog or a sprint—it's only for 20 seconds. If you're indoors on the treadmill, try increasing the speed by at least 1.0 mph or raising the incline by at least 2 percent. On other machines, like a stationary bike or elliptical trainer, increase pedal strokes or resistance by a few points.

MINUTES	INTENSITY	TALK TEST	HEART RATE (OPTIONAL)	RPE
0–3:00	Light (warmup)	Easy conversation	Below VT1	3–4
3:00–13:00	Medium-high	Challenging (short phrases)	10–15 beats above VT1	7–8
13:00–13:20	Very high	Very challenging	15–20 beats above VT1	9
13:20–14:00	Medium-high	Challenging (short phrases)	10–15 beats above VT1	7–8
14:00-14:20	Very high	Very challenging	15–20 beats above VT1	9
14:20–15 :00	Medium-high	Challenging (short phrases)	10–15 beats above VT1	7–8
15:00–15:20	Very high	Very challenging	15–20 beats above VT1	9
15:20–16:00	Medium-high	Challenging (short phrases)	10–15 beats above VT1	7–8
16:00–16:20	Very High	Very challenging	15–20 beats above VT1	9
16:20–17:00	Medium-High	Challenging (short phrases)	10–15 beats above VT1	7–8
17:00–17:20	Very High	Very challenging	15–20 beats above VT1	9
17:20–18:00	Medium-High	Challenging (short phrases)	10–15 beats above VT1	7–8
18:00–18:20	Very High	Very challenging	15–20 beats above VT1	9
18:20 –19:00	Medium-High	Challenging (short phrases)	10–15 beats above VT1	7–8
19:00–19:20	Very High	Very challenging	15–20 beats above VT1	9
19:20–20:00	Medium-High	Challenging (short phrases)	10–15 beats above VT1	7–8
20:00–27:00	Medium High	Challenging (short phrases)	10–15 beats above VT1	7–8
27:00–32:00	Medium	Somewhat challenging	At VT1	5
32:00–35:00	Light (cooldown)	Easy conversation	Below VT1	3–4

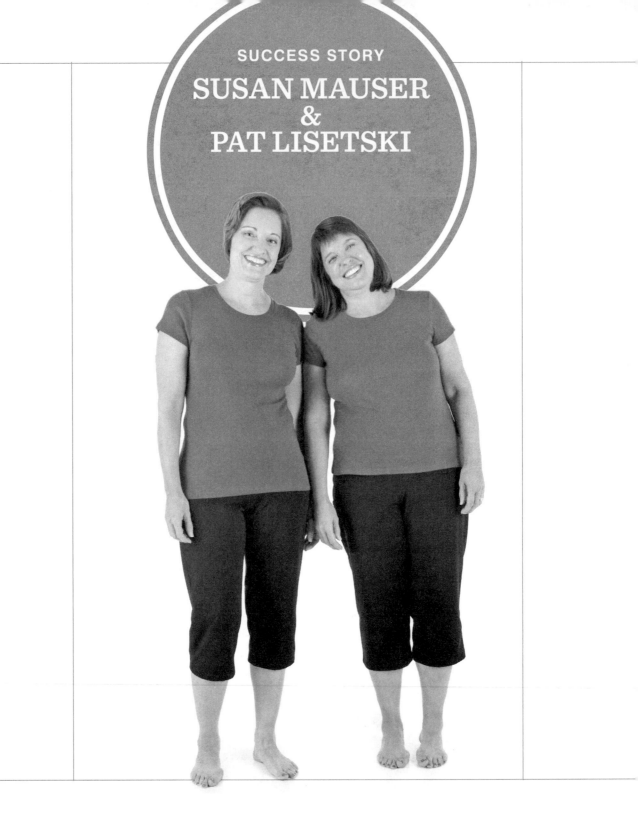

SUCCESS STORY

SUSAN MAUSER & PAT LISETSKI

SUSAN

Age: 45

Height: 5'6"

Pounds lost: 6

Inches lost: $2\frac{3}{4}$

What she's most proud of: "I can keep up with my husband when he goes for a run!"

Favorite foods: Weight Watchers ice cream bars; fat-free Greek yogurt; multigrain pretzels with flaxseed

PAT

Age: 51

Height: 5'4"

Pounds lost: $6\frac{1}{2}$

Inches lost: $4\frac{3}{4}$

What she's most proud of: "I feel younger and stronger."

Favorite foods: Vanilla peach smoothie; fresh veggies with low-fat dressing

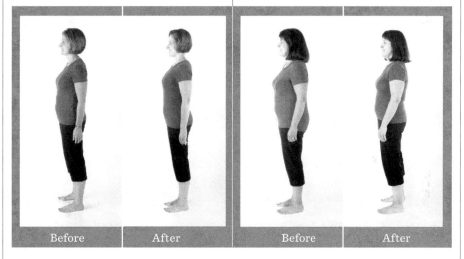

Before   After   Before   After

Sisters Pat Lisetski and Susan Mauser are alike in many ways. They're both middle-school teachers. They like to walk regularly. They're both veterans of many a weight-loss plan, often going on diets at the same time. But while they did a weekly walking workout together and frequently compared notes on fat grams, calories, and points, they never really combined exercise and diet in one set program—and they mostly skipped strength training entirely.

The two signed on to do the Turn Up Your Fat Burn program together, and while they did the circuit workouts and

continued

some of the cardio on their own, they kept up their weekly walks with a third sister, this time doing intervals that included jogging to get their heart rates into their training zones.

"Doing just 35 minutes of run/walk intervals felt like a much better workout than our usual 60-minute power walk," says Susan, who dropped 6 pounds and 1 inch off her waist, plus another 1$\frac{1}{2}$ inches off her hips, in 4 weeks. "When it came time to jog, I began to feel much stronger and less sluggish. And after the workouts, I feel much more energized!"

Adding strength circuits also helped boost results. "The combination of cardio and strength really seemed to work for us," says Pat, who lost 6$\frac{1}{2}$ pounds and 2 inches from her waistline, as well as an inch from her hips, during her 4 weeks on the panel. "I hadn't really done any true weight training for some time or any intervals—we usually just went out and walked. Doing both in one plan made a big difference."

"The strength was a lot less boring than I anticipated," adds Susan. "In the past, I always went from machine to machine, but it never really felt like much of a challenge. With the circuit programs, my heart rate was up, and I was definitely getting a workout!"

Her favorite exercise for developing a firmer core: planks. "I even added a few extras because I really felt like it worked my abs."

For both, the results were measurable and came quickly. "Almost every time I did a pushup in a workout, I could see I was getting stronger," says Pat. "I started out just being able to do about four, then it went to five, then six, then seven!" Her strength has paid off in other ways, too. "It's easier to get off the floor if I'm sitting or even when I'm just squatting down to get something out of a low cupboard. I feel like I have more control of my body. And I don't feel 'old' anymore!"

The workouts and diet also helped Susan control some digestive issues and bloating she's been combating for the past few years. "I think focusing on adding more fiber to my diet was key," says Susan, who often reached for fiber-rich snacks like pretzels with flaxseed, multigrain crackers, almonds, and fruit like Honeycrisp apples. "I had to work on eating more throughout the day so I wouldn't be so hungry later at night."

She notes her weight issue started when she got married about 6 years ago. "I always lived by myself and didn't keep much food at home, but when my husband started to cook for me, the pounds came on." Now, she says, "I feel healthier and more energized. I'm sleeping better, and I'm more confident."

The pair did a 5-K race together, this time running the full distance. "We were going to power walk it but decided to try running instead, and I ran the whole race, coming in at just under my goal of 30 minutes," says Susan, who notes that she hasn't really been a runner since she was in her twenties. "I truly believe the interval training helped get my endurance up to be able to complete the 5-K."

Five months after starting the plan, both Pat and Susan report they've continued to keep up the strength training at least 2 days a week and do the interval (run/walks) at least once a week. "Finding time in life continues to be the struggle, but I haven't given up!" claims Pat. While she says her weight hasn't downshifted dramatically, she's wearing smaller jeans and continues to feel stronger during daily activities. "When I look in the mirror, I notice that my arms seem more developed and my belly looks flatter."

Susan also notes her clothes continue to fit better. "I really notice it in my pants and jeans," she says. "I feel more confident in myself. My stomach seems flatter, and people have told me I look more toned, especially in my upper body."

Both stuck to the 1,600-calorie guidelines and found that their meals and snacks kept them satisfied. "If you eat well, you don't feel hungry," says Pat, who favors lots of fresh veggies with low-fat dressing, plenty of fruit, and a daily yogurt for one of her snacks. "I never felt like I was constantly searching for something to eat."

And while losing inches and pounds has been motivating, Pat says she's also inspired to keep up the exercise for her health. About 2 years ago, she was diagnosed with ductal carcinoma in situ (DCIS), a form of breast cancer that, while not considered life threatening, can increase the risk of developing a more invasive form of the disease. "Exercise can help reduce your cancer risk, so it's definitely something I'm thinking about," notes Pat. "I think of this as just a few minutes I'm investing in myself."

PART IV

Eat Right,
Burn Fat

What Should You Eat?

We've talked a lot so far about the role of exercise in reducing body fat, but if you're serious about losing weight, you can't ignore your diet. You don't have to starve yourself to lose a few inches around your waistline, though. Quite the contrary: If you cut back on calories too drastically, you'll slow your metabolism so your body will want desperately to hold on to every calorie it gets—which can make losing that extra weight even more difficult. Of course, you don't get to binge on pizza, fries, burgers, and sweets. Your body needs the right kind of nutrition to burn fat the best.

We asked Tracy Gensler, MS, RD, a nutritionist specializing in weight loss and sports nutrition, to create an eating plan with enough food and choices to keep you satisfied and ready for action.

"DIET" IS A FOUR-LETTER WORD

Most of us have tried at least one (or maybe a dozen) diets over the years. There are plenty of eating regimens out there to choose from: juice fasts, hot-pepper-and-honey cleansers, ultra-low-fat options, super-high protein plans. So what works?

Research has shown that the type of diet (low-carb, high-carb, low-fat, high-protein) doesn't matter as much as the fact that you're actually watching what you eat. Harvard researchers followed more than 800 adults assigned one of four diets differing in fat, protein, and carb content; during the 2-year study, all the dieters lost about the same amount of weight. The moral of the story: Any reduced-calorie diet can result in meaningful weight loss.

However, not every reduced-calorie diet will keep you happy. Those high-protein/low-carb plans may help you drop a lot of water weight at first, but after a while, you're going to have a dream about swimming in a bowl of pasta. And the super-low-fat programs will make it impossible to navigate a restaurant meal without having to scrape every bit of sauce off your entrée.

We want your experience over the next month—and the months and years to follow—to be positive, not one that will make you want to gnaw off your arm by dinnertime. If you're starving halfway through the afternoon and can't wait to finally attack your pantry, you're going to undo all the gains you've made through the exercise portion of the program. Plus, if you're not properly fueled for the workouts, you won't perform at your best, which will compromise your results.

So our first goal is to keep you energized for the exercises and satisfied all day long. That means providing you with a healthy balance of macronutrients—a balance of about 45 to 50 percent carbs, 20 percent protein, and 30 to 35 percent fat. (Percentages may vary depending on your food choices; for example, if you choose mostly vegetarian meals, you'll get a higher amount of carbohydrates.)

Carbs are important because, as we learned in Chapter 1, they are your body's go-to fuel source when you exercise. Also, the rest of your body—especially your brain—can't function without adequate carbohydrates. Protein plays an important role in hundreds of your body's functions, including helping your muscles rebuild and get stronger after exercise. Fat is vital for everything from fueling workouts and carrying vitamins through the body to helping you feel full longer.

Our second goal is to keep things simple. Let's face it: If you have to prepare elaborate meals with hard-to-find or expensive ingredients, you're probably going to just pick up the phone and order takeout or fall back on your old standbys. We're keeping the meals basic (but still tasty) and easy to prepare. Since real life includes eating out (including fast food), we've even included some popular restaurant items. You'll find these listed in the plan as "on-the-go" options.

Our final goal is to offer a wide variety of delicious choices. Not everyone likes the same kinds of food. Some of us can't stand seafood, others are practically vegetarian, and others are pure carnivores who want a bit of meat at every meal. This program is designed to cover an array of healthy options with a mix of nutrients, so there's a little something for everyone. You'll find everything from fruits and veggies to wraps and salads, and even treats to satisfy your sweet tooth.

THE TURN UP YOUR FAT BURN EATING PLAN

So what *should* you be eating over the next few weeks? That's largely up to you! In the next chapter, we'll provide 2 weeks' worth of meals and snacks—more than 60 in total—giving you plenty of options to choose from over the days and weeks ahead. Each day you'll have three main meals plus two snacks. All of these meals are designed to meet the few overarching principles that will make this plan successful. You can include your own creations, but try to stay within the following guidelines.

Keep within the calorie count

Our goal here is to keep you satisfied without piling on too many calories. The equation is simple: The more calories you consume, the more likely your body will store what it doesn't use through exercise or daily function. **In the plan, you'll be eating about 1,600 calories each day.** The meals and snacks have these approximate calorie counts.

Breakfast: 300 calories

Snack 1: 200 calories

Lunch: 450 calories

Snack 2: 200 calories

Dinner: 450 calories

Total: 1,600 calories

It's important to have at least a rough idea of how many calories you are taking in each day. If you're following the menu and preparing the meals and snacks that Tracy has created, this will be easy, since she's calculated the approximate calorie counts. If you're choosing different foods, you'll need to read the labels or look up the calorie counts. You may get a serious reality check on the number of calories in your meals and in one serving. If you're dining out, keep an eye on your portions—restaurant fare can sometimes pack an entire day's worth of calories in a single meal.

Many of our test panel members said that 1,600 calories a day was a surprisingly satisfying amount, even when they were used to consuming far more calories. "I found I never really got too hungry, even by the end of the day," notes Loretta Marsicano. "I'm someone who used to skip a lot of meals and then binge, but this helped me stay on top of my calorie needs."

Track what you eat

One of the best tools for determining how many calories you're consuming each day is a food log. Numerous studies have shown that dieters who keep tabs on what they eat are more successful at losing weight and keeping it off.

We've provided a few logs beginning on page 341 to help you get started. They'll allow you to take note of everything you eat and drink

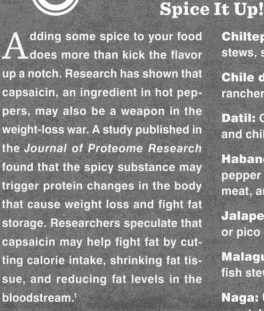

Spice It Up!

Adding some spice to your food does more than kick the flavor up a notch. Research has shown that capsaicin, an ingredient in hot peppers, may also be a weapon in the weight-loss war. A study published in the *Journal of Proteome Research* found that the spicy substance may trigger protein changes in the body that cause weight loss and fight fat storage. Researchers speculate that capsaicin may help fight fat by cutting calorie intake, shrinking fat tissue, and reducing fat levels in the bloodstream.[1]

There are several kinds of spicy peppers. Try adding some heat to your next meal or snack. (The white membrane and seeds are the source of the spiciness, so simply use less of them if the pepper is too piquant for your taste.)

Aji: Use this South American pepper in salsa, ceviche, sauces, or pickled dishes.

Cayenne: Add it, finely chopped, to sauces, stews, soups, or dips.

Chiltepin: Chop it up for soups, stews, salsas or chorizo.

Chile de arbol: Use it in huevos rancheros or fish dishes.

Datil: Great for hot sauce recipes and chili.

Habanero: This all-around chile pepper is ideal for sauces, chili, meat, and seafood dishes.

Jalapeño: Dice and add to salsa or pico de gallo.

Malagueta: Sprinkle into chili or fish stew.

Naga: Use to flavor canning vegetables.

Scotch bonnet: Adds flavor to Jamaican jerk spice and curries.

Rocoto: Commonly known as manzano chile, it's delicious in salsa.

Tabasco: Use as a condiment for any dish needing a little heat. It's especially good in fish dishes.

Thai pepper: Complements kebab-style grilled veggies and meat.

throughout the day. The more days you track, the better the results you'll get. A Kaiser Permanente study of more than 1,600 overweight or obese adults found that those who kept food records at least 6 days a week for 6 months lost about twice as much weight as those who did so once a week or less.[2]

Several free online programs can also be used to keep track of what you eat, including MyPyramidTracker.gov and the free My Health Trackers tool at Prevention.com. Test panel member Lisa Miller says using My Health Trackers really helped her stick with the guidelines: "It kept track of everything for me, and I could just pick foods that I'd already had before so I didn't need to type it all in again. It was sort of like having a nutritionist standing over the table with me."

Watch portion sizes

Over the years, portion sizes have grown along with many of our waistlines. When you're cooking at home, measuring cups and spoons can help you determine how much to eat, but when you're dining out, it can sometimes be hard to measure one serving size. Here's a good trick: Use your hand to guesstimate the proper portion size before you start to eat.

Thumb tip = 1 teaspoon of butter or oil

Full thumb = 1-ounce serving of cheese

Fist = Medium portion of fruit or 1 cup of rice or pasta

Palm (not including fingers) = 4-ounce serving of meat, poultry, or fish

Cupped hand = 1 serving of cereal, pretzels, or chips

A Sweeter Spice

Cinnamon is another spice that can both add flavor and play a role in your bottom line. Research has found that an active compound in cinnamon can increase glucose metabolism (the process of converting glucose to energy) by nearly 20 times. It's also a powerful antioxidant, helping to prevent diseases such as cancer and diabetes.[3] Sprinkle some ground cinnamon on toast or oatmeal, or add a pinch to hot cocoa or baked acorn squash.

Go Nuts!

There was a time when a conscientious dieter would not dare go near a jar of nuts for fear of undoing all of her weight-loss progress. But now we know that, in small amounts, nuts aren't a negative—in fact, they're actually quite helpful when it comes to shedding pounds.

Several major epidemiological and clinical studies have shown that nuts are not associated with weight gain. Researchers speculate that although nuts are relatively energy dense (a half ounce of mixed nuts has about 84 calories), they can keep you satisfied for hours. One study found that among men and women on low-fat diets, those who ate a few ounces of almonds lost about $6\frac{1}{2}$ inches from their waistlines in 6 months—nearly 50 percent more than those who didn't nosh on nuts.[4] There's even some evidence that eating nuts will boost resting energy expenditure, the amount of calories you burn all day.

Nuts can add flavor to your diet in plenty of ways.

Almonds: Great for vegetable salads, with rice or couscous, or in fruit salads.

Cashews: Add to stir-fries and salads.

Macadamia nuts: Flavorful with tropical fruits such as kiwifruit, pineapple, or mango and with mild fish such as cod or tilapia.

Pecans: These sweet nuts are excellent with winter squash such as acorn or butternut. Stir them into muffin or pancake mixes.

Pistachios: Toss into chicken salad and pasta dishes to add a savory crunch.

Eat often—breakfast, lunch, dinner, and snacks

In Chapter 3, we talked about the importance of eating at regular intervals. On this program, there's no shortage of eating opportunities—in fact, you'll be eating at least five times a day, including three meals and two snacks. Eating more frequently will keep you satisfied. We all know how it feels to skip a meal or wait until late in the day to eat: More often than not, the delay's followed by a total binge.

By dividing your food intake among small meals and snacks spaced throughout the day, you'll be less hungry, less likely to grab something utterly unhealthy, and a lot less cranky. You will also have enough fuel in your system to keep you going through your workouts. If you start a workout already feeling hungry or light-headed, it's going to be difficult to perform at your best and get all that you can out of each circuit or interval.

There's another reason to eat more often: When you eat, you burn calories digesting the food and transporting nutrients throughout your body. Digestion uses 10 percent of the calories you take in every day.

Not everyone likes to eat a lot in the morning, but we strongly recommend eating breakfast every day. The rest of the timing is largely up to you. You can keep one snack as a midmorning meal, or save one snack for dessert after dinner. You know what works best for you and your cravings. But try not to go more than 4 or 5 hours between meals, or your blood sugar levels will get too low, and you'll be more likely to lose control of your eating. Panelist Cindy Wenrich notes that eating more frequently helped level off her between-meal snacking: "Because I was having smaller meals and snacks every few hours, I never got too hungry. I'm going to keep eating this way from now on!"

Since not all of us are built the same way, you may find yourself needing or wanting an additional snack. Tall women (over 5'8") require more calories because they have more body mass. Men require more calories because they have more muscle mass, which results in a faster metabolism. So if you fall into either of these categories, add one of the special 300-calorie snacks if you get hungry. The rest of us can add a third 200-calorie snack if needed, but keep in mind that it will bring your daily calorie intake to 1,800 to 1,900.

Have at least 25 grams of fiber a day

On our plan, you'll consume at least 8 grams of fiber with each breakfast, lunch, and dinner and at least 2 grams with each snack. Why the high-fiber fix? Research shows that adults who have higher intakes of fiber are leaner. Including fiber-rich foods in your diet every day can help you maintain body weight or prevent excess weight gain over time.

A German study of nearly 25,000 middle-aged men and women

Hitting the Bars

When you're out and about or just don't have time to put together a snack, sometimes it's easiest to grab an energy bar. There are certainly many to choose from: crunchy, sweet, nutty, flaky. Which are the best to pick? Follow these simple rules.

○ The bar should have no more than 2 grams of saturated fat and at least 3 grams fiber.

○ If you want the bar to count as a snack, make sure it has 200 calories or fewer (300 calories if you're adding the bonus snack).

○ Look for whole grains on the ingredients list. Whole wheat, oats, nuts (any type), or fruit should be the first or second ingredient.

○ Keep processing to a minimum: The fewer ingredients the better. Choose a bar with mostly whole foods in the ingredients list, including dried fruit, grains, and nuts.

○ Don't limit yourself to bars. Many snack foods are easy to assemble, just as portable, and a lot less expensive than an energy bar. Try whole wheat bread spread with peanut butter and sprinkled with raisins or a piece of fruit with a couple of tablespoons of nuts.

found that those who followed a diet rich in fiber and low in fat either maintained their weight or were less likely to gain as much weight as those who ate a low-fiber, high-fat diet over a 4-year period—a more than 16-pound difference in body weight between those with the highest fiber intake and those with the lowest.[5] Researchers at Tufts University found that choosing whole grains over refined can help fight belly fat. The study of more than 2,800 men and women found that those who had three or more servings of whole grains a day and less than one serving of refined grains had about 10 percent less visceral adipose tissue or belly fat. Those who ate both whole grains and refined foods didn't experience the same belly-flattening benefits.[6]

Why does fiber play such an important role in weight loss or maintenance? For starters, high-fiber foods usually take longer to chew, which means you're not scarfing down your meal. Your body has time to fully register that you're satisfied, so you're less likely to overeat. Fiber also "bulks up" a meal so you'll stay fuller longer. Plus, high-fiber foods tend to be less dense in energy, which means they're lower in calories.

The USDA recommends a minimum of 25 grams of fiber per day for women and 38 grams per day for men under age 51, and 21 grams for women and 30 grams for men over age 51.[7] On this plan you'll get no fewer than 34 and sometimes as many as 48 grams per day.

How can you get more fiber in your diet? Besides following the menu and meal ideas in this chapter, here are a few simple ideas to help you get your fill.

○ Begin each lunch and dinner with a veggie-packed soup or salad.

○ Choose whole grain bread, crackers, pasta, and cereal. Look for the word *whole* in the ingredients list.

○ Have a snack of air-popped popcorn; 3 cups has 3½ grams of fiber and fewer than 100 calories.

○ Go meatless for dinner at least once a week: Have a fiber-rich vegetarian meal such as rice and beans with vegetables or a stir-fry with mixed vegetables like broccoli, cauliflower, and carrots, plus edamame.

○ Eat whole fruit. OJ may be tasty, but a whole orange has five times more fiber than a glass of juice and only half the calories.

○ Fill out your meal. Add fresh or frozen vegetables to soups and sauces. Try throwing some spinach or broccoli into spaghetti sauce, or make turkey chili with carrots, peppers, and beans.

Have one magnesium-rich meal per day

Magnesium is a mighty mineral that many of us ignore. According to the USDA, about 60 percent of US adults don't consume the recommended dietary allowance of 320 milligrams for women over the age of 30 and

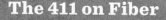

The 411 on Fiber

Dietary fibers are all the parts of plant foods that you can't digest. We use *fiber* as a catch-all term, but there are really two kinds of fiber: soluble and insoluble. Ideally, you should get some of both kinds of fiber in your diet.

Soluble fiber (so named because it dissolves in water) binds to fatty substances and carries them out as waste. It helps regulate blood sugars so you stay fuller longer, and it also helps lower LDL ("bad") cholesterol and control blood sugar levels. Soluble fiber is found in foods like oats, peas, beans, apples, oranges, grapefruit, carrots, and barley. (This is not to be confused with dissolving fiber powders that you can buy to add to food—we do not recommend these as substitutes for fiber obtained directly from food.)

Insoluble fiber (which does not dissolve in water) is sort of like a big broom for your digestive tract. It helps sweep waste through your colon to prevent constipation and keep you regular. Insoluble fiber is found in whole wheat products, nuts, and many vegetables.

420 milligrams for men over 30 (the numbers are slightly lower for people age 19 to 30).[8] That's too bad, because magnesium plays an important role in exercise and diet, not to mention numerous other vital functions. It's needed for more than 300 biochemical reactions in the body, helping to maintain normal muscle and nerve function, a steady heart rate, a healthy immune system, and strong bones. Magnesium helps create ATP, the main source of fuel when muscles contract. It aids absorption of calcium and can lower blood pressure. There's evidence that a diet rich in magnesium could reduce a person's risk of metabolic syndrome, a cluster of health problems (obesity, high blood pressure, high cholesterol) that can lead to diabetes and heart disease.

Magnesium may also play an important role in decreasing the risk of type 2 diabetes. According to the Nurses' Health Study and the Health Professionals' Follow-Up Study of more than 170,000 health professionals, men and women with lower magnesium intakes had a greater risk of developing diabetes.[9] One theory is that a deficiency in magnesium can cause insulin to function poorly, which may increase blood-sugar levels and the storage of fat.

Luckily, lots of healthy (and tasty) foods have an abundance of magnesium, including spinach, black beans, salmon, scallops, tuna, almonds, cashews, and brown rice. (For a complete list, see "Maximum Magnesium," below.) Just be careful to watch the calorie count, since some of these foods (especially nuts and grains) can be calorie dense.

In the Turn Up Your Fat Burn eating plan, many of the lunch and dinner options provide a boost of magnesium. Alternatively, assemble your own magnesium-rich meals by including one full portion of any of the foods listed in the chart. Bonus: Most of these foods are also very good sources of fiber.

Note that the cooked amounts of foods don't include any added fat. Feel free to use some olive oil or other fat in preparation, but keep your lunch or dinner meal to about 450 calories to stay in line with the plan.

Maximum Magnesium

FOOD	PORTION	CALORIES	GRAMS FIBER	PERCENTAGE DAILY VALUE OF MAGNESIUM	MILLIGRAMS MAGNESIUM
Spinach, chopped, cooked	¾ cup	31	3	29	117
Swiss chard, cooked	¾ cup	26	3	28	113
Almonds, whole, dry roasted	¼ cup	212	4	25	99
Brazil nuts	3 tablespoons	172	2	25	99
Edamame, shelled, cooked	1 cup	244	10	25	99
Sesame seeds, dried whole	3 tablespoons	155	3	25	95
Lima beans, cooked	¾ cup	157	7	24	94

FOOD	PORTION	CALORIES	GRAMS FIBER	PERCENTAGE DAILY VALUE OF MAGNESIUM	MILLIGRAMS MAGNESIUM
Pumpkin or squash seed kernels, dried	2 tablespoons	94	1	23	93
Navy beans, cooked	¾ cup	222	10	23	92
Scallops, cooked	6 ounces	180	0	23	92
Halibut, cooked	3 ounces	119	0	23	91
Cashews	¼ cup	197	1	22	89
Quinoa, cooked	¾ cup	167	4	22	89
Sunflower seed kernels, dried	3 tablespoons	162	3	22	88
Tempeh, cooked	4 ounces	222	4	22	87
Brown rice, cooked	1 cup	220	4	21	86
Buckwheat groats, cooked	1 cup	155	5	21	86
Pine nuts or pignolia	¼ cup	232	1	22	86
Black beans, canned, no salt added	1 cup	218	17	21	84
Quinoa, dry	¼ cup	156	3	21	84
Flaxseed, ground	3 tablespoons	112	6	20	82
Pinto, calico, or red Mexican beans, cooked	1 cup	182	9	20	81
Millet, cooked	¾ cup	214	2	20	79

Have some fat—but make it the right kind

All fat isn't bad—in fact, some fats, in moderation, can be downright good for you! The key is to distinguish good fats from bad.

Let's start with the bad guys. There's no doubt that too much saturated fat is unhealthy. According to the American Heart Association, saturated fat is the main dietary cause of high blood cholesterol and a primary culprit in heart disease. This plan limits saturated fat to less than 10 percent of total daily calories to help control your blood cholesterol.

Trans fats are like saturated fats' evil double. These fats (created by heating liquid vegetable oil in the presence of hydrogen gas) make foods more stable, easier to transport, and less likely to break down when heated repeatedly (as in frying fast foods), but they're even worse than other fats at raising LDL ("bad") cholesterol levels and lowering HDL ("good") cholesterol.

Even a small amount of trans fat can be dangerous. According to a study published in the *New England Journal of Medicine,* for every extra 2 percent of calories from trans fats consumed each day (about the amount in a medium order of fries), the risk of coronary heart disease increases 23 percent.[10] Many restaurants and food companies have worked to cut down the amount of trans fats in their products, and the FDA requires food labels to list whether there are any trans fats in products, but there are still lots of trans fats in processed foods and restaurant offerings.

Now for the good guys. Unsaturated fats can have a positive effect on your health. There are two primary types of unsaturated fat: monounsaturated and polyunsaturated (each has different chemical structures). Unsaturated fats are found in olive, canola, and sesame oil, as well as in many types of fish and nuts like almonds and pecans. An abundance of research has shown that unsaturated fats improve cholesterol levels, reduce inflammation, lower the risk of heart disease, and even improve brain function. The Nurses' Health Study found that replacing 80 calories of carbohydrates with 80 calories of polyunsaturated or monounsaturated fats lowered the risk of heart disease by about 30 to 40 percent.[11]

Two types of polyunsaturated fat—omega-3 and omega-6 fatty acids—have gotten a lot of buzz for their health and even weight-loss benefits. Omega-3s are found in foods like walnuts, flaxseed, and fatty fish like salmon. Most of us probably don't get as much omega-3 in our diets as we should. Try to eat at least one food rich in omega-3 fatty acids each day, whether that's a fish dish like salmon, a handful of walnuts, or something cooked with canola oil. When these fats were added to a reduced-calorie diet in a study, participants lost about 2.2 more pounds after 4 weeks than those who were on a similar diet without the added fats.[12]

Omega-6 fatty acids (found in safflower and corn oils, among others) are widely consumed in the United States. While omega-6s can help ease aches and clear up acne and other skin conditions, there's some concern that we get too much of it, which can cause bloating, high blood pressure, and other health problems.

Here's a list of the different kinds of fats found in some of our most common food choices.

Saturated fats

Beef, veal, lamb, pork, and poultry with skin

Dairy: butter, cream, milk, cheese and other dairy products made from whole and 2% milk

Palm oil and palm kernel oil (often called tropical oils), cocoa butter

Trans fats

Foods with the label "partially hydrogenated vegetable oils"

Monounsaturated fats

Canola, peanut, and olive oil

Avocados

Almonds, hazelnuts, and pecans

Pumpkin and sesame seeds

Polyunsaturated fats

Sunflower, corn, soybean, and flaxseed oils

Walnuts and flaxseed

Fish

For a well-balanced diet that minimizes the bad fats and promotes the good ones, follow these guidelines.

○ Choose fruits, vegetables, and fat-free and low-fat dairy foods.

○ Avoid processed foods with partially hydrogenated or hydrogenated vegetable oils in the ingredients list.

○ Use spreads with "0 g trans fat" on the Nutrition Facts label.

○ Avoid fried foods, french fries, doughnuts, cookies, muffins, pies, and cakes.

Drink up

In Chapter 3, you learned why it helps to drink 8 to 10 glasses of cold water a day. Water is crucial to keeping you healthy and ready for action. Drink it cold and you may even boost your metabolism a bit, according to research. A recent study from Virginia Tech also found that subjects who drank ½ liter (about 2 cups) of water before each meal lost about 4½ more pounds over 12 weeks than those who didn't drink up.[13]

Of course, water isn't the only healthy beverage. Tea—beloved around the world for centuries—has been garnering attention lately for its role in weight loss. Research shows that both green and black tea (they actually come from the same plant; the different color comes from the drying process) contain antioxidant substances called catechins that can boost weight loss and provide many health benefits.

One recent study from the *Journal of Nutrition* found that overweight and obese men and women who did about 30 minutes of moderate exercise a day and drank a daily beverage fortified with the same amount of catechins found in about 3 cups of green tea for 12 weeks lost nearly 8 times more abdominal fat than those who exercised and drank an ordinary caffeinated beverage.[14] Other research showed that an extract found in black tea helped prevent weight gain among rats fed a high-fat diet.[15]

Can't give up your coffee? That's okay. Your morning cup isn't bad for your health, according to the Nurses' Health Study and Health Professionals' Follow-Up Study, which found that even those who drank up to 6 cups of java a day had no increased risk of death from any cause, including cardiovascular disease or cancer.[16] And the caffeine in coffee (and tea) may help suppress your appetite and even boost your metabolism slightly. Just make sure you account for added sugar, milk, or cream, which can more than double the calories in the cup. Of course, caffeine isn't for everyone, especially if you're on certain blood pressure medications or have a heart condition. If you're concerned about consuming too much caffeine, check with your doctor, or just order decaf.

What about wine, beer, and other adult libations? You're making a commitment to yourself to eat smart, live healthy, and improve your fitness for 1 month. Alcohol can undermine all three goals. Alcoholic beverages are not only frequently high in calories but can lead to unhealthy eating habits. So try to avoid alcoholic beverages for the next 4 weeks. Opt for sparkling water with a wedge of lemon or lime when you're at a party or social gathering.

Eat breakfast

Beginning your day with a healthy breakfast is one of the best ways to stay on track for weight loss. When you skip breakfast, you tend to make up for it later in the day. Numerous studies have shown that eating breakfast is key to losing or maintaining weight.

Consider adding an egg to your morning meal. Several studies have shown that eating an egg for breakfast can help keep your weight in check. One found that women who ate two eggs for breakfast at least 5 days a week for 8 weeks lost 65 percent more weight and reduced their waistlines by 80 percent more, compared with those who had a bagel breakfast with the same amount of calories.[17]

FREQUENTLY ASKED QUESTIONS

Before we move on to the specifics of the plan, we wanted to address a couple of the questions you may have.

I'm starving by the end of the day. Isn't there anything else I can eat?

Tracy designed this plan to keep you satisfied, so extreme hunger shouldn't be a problem. But if you're on the taller/larger/bigger side, you may find yourself wanting a little more during the day. Add the optional 300-calorie snack whenever you think you need it (you can also try a 200-calorie one instead). That should be enough to keep you going! Remember to space your meals and snacks out so your hunger levels don't get too out of control.

Do I have to follow the meal plan exactly?

Our focus is more on exercise than diet, but what you eat will definitely affect your results. You don't have to eat each and every meal on the plan, but at least get a sense of portion sizes and calorie content of the suggested meals and snacks. If you follow the guidelines—consuming an average of 1,600 calories a day (including 25 grams of fiber and one magnesium-rich food) by eating three meals plus two snacks and drinking lots of water—you should enjoy the same great results as our test panelists who followed the meal plan.

"I dropped two pants sizes!"

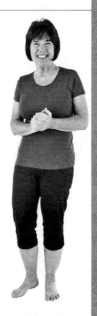

At the beginning of the summer, Leslie Tang's oldest daughter gave her a pair of size 8 capris she couldn't wait to put on. Unfortunately, she couldn't zip them up. "I realized I really was more like a size 12," she says.

Leslie had been gaining weight steadily over the past few years, especially since having a hysterectomy. "I never had much of a belly before, but after the surgery, I definitely noticed more weight gain in my midsection," she says.

Leslie started watching portion sizes and increased her activity, walking her two dogs for up to 2 miles every day. The weight started coming off, but after a while, "I hit a plateau," says Leslie, who started her 4-week program at nearly 163 pounds. "No matter what I did, I couldn't get below 160."

Doing intervals helped boost her overall conditioning, while the strength routine made a difference in her definition. "My waist definitely seems thinner, and my abdomen looks flatter and feels firmer," she says. After a month on the plan, she dropped 6 pounds and 2½ inches, including 1½ inches off her waistline.

The workouts also gave her a much-needed energy boost both at work and with her family: "I went hiking with my kids recently, and it was absolutely no problem to do the whole hilly trail."

She found that having a list of healthy foods to choose from kept her on track with her diet and portion sizes and says her whole family is now in on the act. "Every time I make something now, my youngest daughter wants to try it! We're introducing a lot of new foods in our house."

And those capris? They now fit perfectly. "I'm fitting into a lot of clothes I couldn't get into before. I'm hoping to eventually get down to a 6."

CHAPTER **11**

The Turn Up Your Fat Burn Eating Plan

Now that you have the basic framework for what you should be eating over the next 4 weeks, it's time to dig in!

We've created a plan that is both extremely flexible and easy to follow. There's something for everyone—meat lovers, vegetarians, and everyone in between. It's all about picking and choosing what you like the best, while still keeping within the simple Turn Up Your Fat Burn eating plan guidelines. Pick the meals and snacks that sound good and fit with your tastes and schedule—it's as easy as that. If you still don't see anything here that you like, follow the handy "Build Your Own Meal" chart on page 225, which will allow you to customize your choices.

All of the breakfasts are interchangeable. So are

the snack options, so you can go sweet or savory, depending on your mood. Lunches and dinners are a little more substantial; you can switch those around as well and still be satisfied.

Following are more than 60 choices for healthy, tasty breakfasts, lunches, dinners, and snacks. Most of the meals are single servings and can be prepared in 30 minutes or less. If you're cooking for your whole family or have a little more time to prepare your food, check out the additional yummy Turn Up Your Fat Burn recipes in Chapter 12.

THREE EASY RULES TO FOLLOW

Rule 1. Eat a total of about 1,600 calories a day. Try to spread them throughout the day: a breakfast of about 300 calories, lunch and dinner of about 450 calories each, and two 200-calorie snacks. **Option:** Women over 5′8″ and all men can opt to add a third 300-calorie snack to meet their nutritional needs.

Rule 2. Eat at least 25 grams of fiber per day. The meals described here include 8 grams of fiber (breakfast, lunch, and dinner), while the snacks all have at least 2 grams. If you're creating your own meals and snacks, try to follow the same fiber guidelines. The list of High-Fiber Favorites on the opposite page can help you put together delicious high-fiber meals to your taste. Keep in mind, though, that different brands may vary in the amount of fiber included. (See page 190 for more information on fiber.)

Rule 3. Include at least one magnesium-rich food a day. Each of the dinners on the plan and each lunch or dinner recipe feature a food high in magnesium. Check out the "Maximum Magnesium" list on page 194 to see what works for you (some of these foods also fulfill your fiber requirement).

High-Fiber Favorites

FOOD	SERVING SIZE	GRAMS FIBER
Black beans, cooked	1 cup	16
Lentils, cooked	1 cup	16
Split peas, cooked	1 cup	16
Vegetarian baked beans	1 cup	10.5
Artichoke, cooked	1 medium	10
Lima beans, cooked	1 cup	9.5
Peas, cooked	1 cup	9
Raspberries	1 cup	8
Barley, pearled, cooked	1 cup	6
Spaghetti, whole wheat (cooked)	1 cup	6
Bran flakes	¾ cup	5.5
Pear (with skin)	1 medium	5.5
Oat bran muffin	1 medium	5
Apple (with skin)	1 medium	4.5
Brown rice, cooked	1 cup	4
Brussels sprouts, cooked	1 cup	4
Oatmeal, regular or instant, cooked	1 cup	4
Sunflower seeds	¼ cup	4
Sweet corn, cooked	1 cup	4
Banana	1 medium	3
Orange	1 medium	3
Strawberries	1 cup	3
Almonds	2 tablespoons	2
Broccoli, steamed	1 cup	2
Microwave popcorn	3 cups	1.5

BREAKFASTS

Choose any of these delicious breakfast ideas. Some are perfect for those busy days when you have to get out of the house quickly, while others are ideal for a leisurely weekend morning. All have about 300 calories per serving and at least 8 grams of fiber.

Cereals and Grains

MILANO CEREAL BOWL

Combine ½ cup fat-free Greek yogurt, ¾ cup cereal (pick one with at least 6 grams of fiber in 100 calories' worth, such as Kashi Good Friends), 4 chopped dried figs, and 1 teaspoon agave nectar or honey. Grate ⅛ teaspoon lemon peel over the top.

Total: 299 calories, 0 grams saturated fat, 10 grams fiber

MUESLI

Combine ½ cup fat-free Greek yogurt; ¼ teaspoon each vanilla extract, honey, and cinnamon; ½ cup sliced strawberries; ¼ cup raw steel-cut oats; 1 tablespoon chopped walnuts; and 1 tablespoon ground flaxseed.

Total: 294 calories, 1 gram saturated fat, 8 grams fiber

PECAN OATMEAL

Have 1 cup cooked oatmeal; ½ large baked sweet potato, mashed; and 1 tablespoon pecans.

Total: 290 calories, 1 gram saturated fat, 8 grams fiber

RASPBERRY PANCAKE

In a bowl, whisk together 6 ounces fat-free Greek yogurt, 1 egg, 2 egg whites (or ¼ cup egg substitute), 2 tablespoons whole wheat flour, 1 tablespoon agave nectar or honey, and ⅛ teaspoon salt. Coat a skillet with cooking spray and warm it over medium heat for 1 minute. Make a 3" pancake, cook for 1 to 2 minutes, flip and cook for 1 minute, and remove to a plate. Repeat. Top one pancake with ¾ cup raspberries, 1 tablespoon light maple syrup, and 1½ tablespoons pecans. Save the other pancake for another meal such as the Raspberry Pancake snack on page 216.

Total: 291 calories, 2 grams saturated fat, 8 grams fiber

Egg Dishes

EGG SANDWICH

In a bowl, whisk 2 egg whites, then add 1 tablespoon each chopped green bell pepper and chopped red bell pepper. Heat 1 teaspoon olive oil in a skillet over medium heat and cook the mixture, stirring, until the eggs are set. Place on a toasted whole wheat English muffin and top with two ½"-thick slices of tomato. Serve with 1 medium sliced pear or apple.

Total: 298 calories, 1 gram saturated fat, 15 grams fiber

TAKE-ALONG EGG WRAP

Spread a whole wheat wrap (about 100 calories and 5 grams fiber, such as Flat Out) with 1 tablespoon hummus and top with 1 sliced hard-cooked egg. Serve with 1 banana.

Total: 308 calories, 2 grams saturated fat, 11 grams fiber

VEGGIE SCRAMBLED EGGS AND CRACKERS

Heat ½ teaspoon olive oil in a skill over medium heat. Cook 2 tablespoons chopped onion, stirring, until softened. In a bowl, mix ½ cup spinach leaves, 3 egg whites, ½ teaspoon dried parsley, and ½ teaspoon dried basil. Add to the skillet and cook, stirring, until the eggs are set. On the side, have 1 apple and 8 crackers (120 calories' worth with at least 4 grams fiber, such as Dr. Kracker Organic and Artisan Baked Snackers).

Total: 288 calories, 2 grams saturated fat, 8 grams fiber

Cheesy and Nutty Dishes

CHEESY POLENTA AND BERRIES

Heat 2 teaspoons olive oil in a skillet over medium heat. Cook three ½" slices precooked polenta (from a tube) for 3 minutes. Flip and top each slice with ⅓ ounce 75% reduced-fat Cheddar cheese. Cook for 3 minutes, then transfer to a plate. Top with 1 cup blackberries and drizzle with 1 teaspoon honey.

Total: 293 calories, 3 grams saturated fat, 9 grams fiber

CHEESY ENGLISH MUFFIN

Toast a whole wheat English muffin. Spread with ½ ounce goat cheese and top with 3 strips roasted red pepper from a jar. Serve with 2 kiwifruit, sliced.

Total: 291 calories, 3 grams saturated fat, 10 grams fiber

BAGEL WITH TOMATO AND CHEESE

Slice 1 whole wheat bagel (with about 240 calories and at least 7 grams fiber). Top with 1 slice 2% reduced-fat cheese, any flavor, and 2 thick slices of tomato.

Total: 301 calories, 2 grams saturated fat, 8 grams fiber

PEAR WRAP

Spread a whole wheat wrap (about 100 calories and 5 grams fiber, such as Flat Out) with 1 tablespoon almond butter or peanut butter. Top with 1 large pear, thinly sliced. Roll up. Heat in a microwave oven on high for 20 to 30 seconds.

Total: 297 calories, 1 gram saturated fat, 14 grams fiber

TOAST WITH PEANUT BUTTER AND BANANA

Toast 2 slices whole wheat bread (about 80 calories and at least 3 grams fiber per slice). Spread each slice with 2 teaspoons peanut butter and top with ¼ small banana (save the rest for an afternoon snack).

Total: 296 calories, 2 grams saturated fat, 8 grams fiber

LUNCH OR DINNER CHOICES

The lunches and dinners on the Turn Up Your Fat Burn eating plan are designed to be interchangeable. Some people like a heartier midday meal, while others would rather savor supper toward the end of the day. Pick the meals you like the best; they're all about 450 calories, with at least 8 grams of fiber (most are also a rich source of magnesium). We've added magnesium amounts to the nutritional information in this section so you can track that, if you'd like.

Scrumptious Salads

TACO SALAD

In a small bowl, toss together 3 tablespoons crumbled reduced-fat feta cheese, 1 tablespoon balsamic vinegar, 1 teaspoon olive oil, ⅛ teaspoon chili powder, and ⅛ teaspoon ground red pepper. In another bowl, combine 4 cups shredded romaine, ½ cup thinly sliced red bell pepper, ⅓ cup low-sodium canned kidney beans (rinsed and drained), 4 tablespoons salsa, 1 tablespoon balsamic vinegar, and 1½ teaspoons olive oil. Top the salad with the feta cheese mixture and 1 ounce baked tortilla chips.

Total: 444 calories, 4 grams saturated fat, 13 grams fiber, 41 mg magnesium

SPINACH STRAWBERRY SALAD

Prepare ¾ cup cooked amount wild rice according to package directions. Combine 4 cups spinach leaves with 1 cup sliced strawberries, 3 tablespoons pecans, and 3 tablespoons raspberry vinaigrette. Serve with the hot wild rice on the side.

Total: 456 calories, 3 grams saturated fat, 10 grams fiber, 178 mg magnesium

HEARTY ANTIPASTO SALAD

Cook 1 cup frozen lima beans and allow to cool. In a bowl, combine the lima beans, 2 cups shredded romaine, 3 tablespoons reduced-fat shredded mozzarella cheese, 2 ounces reduced-sodium ham, 1 chopped tomato, 5 large black or green olives, and 3 tablespoons reduced-fat Italian salad dressing (90 calories' worth).

Total: 447 calories, 4 grams saturated fat, 12 grams fiber, 143 mg magnesium

TUNA AND GOLDEN RAISINS

Combine 4 ounces chunk light tuna packed in canola oil (not drained) with 1 tablespoon white vinegar and 2 tablespoons golden or brown raisins. (If the tuna is packed in water, rinse and drain well, then add 2 teaspoons olive or canola oil.) Serve with 1 sliced red, orange, or yellow bell pepper; 8 baby carrots; and 2 whole wheat crackers such as Wasa brand (or 90 calories' worth with at least 4 grams fiber).

Total: 447 calories, 2 grams saturated fat, 10 grams fiber, 59 mg magnesium

SALMON CAESAR SALAD

Combine 3 cups romaine, 1 tablespoon grated Parmesan cheese, 3 ounces (palm-size) broiled salmon, and 1 tablespoon Caesar dressing. Serve with 2 small whole wheat rolls (1.5 ounces for both).

Total: 456 calories, 4 grams saturated fat, 8 grams fiber, 100 mg magnesium

SPINACH SALAD WITH SALMON

Combine 3 cups spinach leaves and 1 cup sliced strawberries. Top with 3 ounces (palm-size) broiled salmon. Dress with 2 teaspoons olive oil and a splash of vinegar. Serve with a baseball-size portion of steamed wild rice.

Total: 459 calories, 3 grams saturated fat, 8 grams fiber, 100 mg magnesium

Savory Sandwiches and Soups

GRILLED CHEESE AND NUTTY TOMATO SOUP

Heat a skillet over low to medium heat. Spread 2 slices whole wheat bread (each 80 calories and about 2 grams fiber) with 4 teaspoons light trans-free spread. Lay 1 slice spread side down in the skillet. Top with 2 slices Cheddar-flavored soy cheese or 1 slice 2% Cheddar cheese and the second slice of bread. Cook for 4 to 5 minutes, or until lightly browned. Flip and repeat on the other side. Heat 1 cup low-sodium tomato soup in a bowl in a microwave oven on high for about 1 minute. Top the soup with 2 tablespoons unsalted soy nuts.

Total: 453 calories, 2 grams saturated fat, 11 grams fiber, 17 mg magnesium

COOL CUCUMBER AVOCADO SANDWICH

Mash 1 ripe Hass avocado with 2 tablespoons salsa, 1 teaspoon olive oil, 2 teaspoons lemon juice, and 3 or 4 shakes of ground red pepper, if desired. Thinly slice 1 cucumber. Top 2 slices of whole wheat bread (80 calories and at least 3 grams fiber per slice) with half of the avocado mixture and one-quarter of the cucumber slices. Serve with the rest of the avocado mixture mixed with another one-quarter of the sliced cucumber. (Save the rest of the cucumber for an afternoon snack on another day.)

Total: 459 calories, 4 grams saturated fat, 15 grams fiber, 59 mg magnesium

CORN AND BLACK BEAN POCKETS

Cook 2 tablespoons frozen corn. Fill 2 medium whole wheat pitas (6" diameter, about 120 calories and 3 grams fiber each) with the corn, 3 tablespoons canned low-sodium black beans, 2 tablespoons salsa, 1½ tablespoons reduced-sodium shredded Cheddar cheese, and ¼ cup shredded romaine.

Total: 446 calories, 4 grams saturated fat, 12 grams fiber, 111 mg magnesium

TURKEY SANDWICH WITH COLESLAW

Combine ¼ cup chopped tomato, 1 teaspoon olive oil, 1 tablespoon balsamic vinegar, and ¼ teaspoon dried basil or 1 teaspoon fresh. Top 2 slices whole wheat bread (80 calories and at least 2 grams fiber per slice) with 4 ounces no-salt-added sliced turkey breast. Top with the tomato mixture. Combine ½ cup each shredded green and red cabbage, ¼ cup grated carrots, and 2 tablespoons reduced-fat coleslaw dressing (or use 1¼ cups prepared coleslaw mix).

Total: 456 calories, 3 grams saturated fat, 8 grams fiber, 19 mg magnesium

CURRIED TUNA PITA

In a small bowl, whisk together 1 tablespoon chopped fresh cilantro, 1 table-spoon fat-free sour cream, 1 tablespoon light mayonnaise, ½ teaspoon lime juice, and a pinch each of curry powder, ground coriander, and salt. In another bowl, combine 4 ounces well-drained water-packed chunk light tuna, 2 small thinly sliced radishes, and 1 tablespoon chopped onion. Toss with the sour cream mixture and top with 1 tablespoon cashews. Serve with one 8" whole wheat pita and half of a large pear.

Total: 451 calories, 2 grams saturated fat, 8 grams fiber, 99 mg magnesium

Hearty Vegetarian Entrées

FIERY EDAMAME

Prepare ¼ cup cooked amount brown rice according to package directions. Toss 1¼ cups cooked edamame, 2 teaspoons sesame oil, ½ teaspoon ground red pepper (or to taste), and 1 small chopped chile pepper. Add the rice. Serve warm or chilled.

Total: 456 calories, 4 grams saturated fat, 14 grams fiber, 33 mg magnesium

DILL-TOPPED VEGGIE BURGER WITH SWEET POTATO FRIES

In a microwave oven, heat 1 veggie burger (about 100 calories). Fill one 2-ounce whole wheat hamburger roll with 4 tablespoons chopped avocado, ¼ cup fat-free Greek yogurt mixed with 1 teaspoon fresh dill or ½ teaspoon dried, and 4 slices cucumber. Serve with 1 cup baked frozen sweet potato fries (about 100 calories' worth, such as Alexia or Hain brand).

Total: 442 calories, 2 grams saturated fat, 14 grams fiber, 91 mg magnesium

CASHEW COUSCOUS

Prepare ½ cup cooked amount whole wheat couscous according to package directions. Heat ¾ teaspoon sesame oil in a skillet over medium heat. Cook ¼ cup cashews and ½ teaspoon ground red pepper, stirring, for 90 seconds. Toss the couscous with the cashew mixture, 1½ tablespoons dried currants, and 1 teaspoon each fresh parsley, sage, and basil or ½ teaspoon dried.

Total: 452 calories, 4 grams saturated fat, 8 grams fiber, 109 mg magnesium

COUSCOUS WITH TOMATOES, CHICKPEAS, AND BRAZIL NUTS

Heat 1½ teaspoons olive oil in a saucepan over medium heat. Cook 3 tablespoons whole wheat couscous, stirring, for 2 to 3 minutes. Add ⅓ cup low-sodium chicken broth, heat to boiling, immediately reduce heat to low, cover, and simmer for 10 to 12 minutes, or until all the water is absorbed. Allow to cool.

Toss the couscous with 1 pint (about 12 ounces) halved grape or cherry tomatoes, 2 teaspoons fresh basil, and ¾ ounce Brazil nuts (about 5), chopped.
Total: 445 calories, 4 grams saturated fat, 8 grams fiber, 77 mg magnesium

COLORFUL CHICKPEA STEW

Heat 2 teaspoons olive oil in a saucepan over low to medium heat. Cook ½ cup shredded carrot, stirring frequently, for 3 to 4 minutes, or until softened. Add 1 cup low-sodium canned chickpeas and ⅛ teaspoon curry powder and cook for 1 to 2 minutes. Transfer to a serving bowl. Mix in 1 tablespoon fresh parsley and 2 teaspoons lemon juice. Serve with 2 cups mixed baby greens topped with 2 tablespoons honey mustard dressing (about 80 calories' worth).
Total: 451 calories, 2 grams saturated fat, 11 grams fiber, 107 mg magnesium

Meat and Poultry Dishes

BEEF ITALIANO

Prepare 1 cup cooked amount brown rice brown rice according to package directions. Heat 1½ teaspoons olive oil in a skillet over medium heat. Cook 3 ounces 95% lean ground beef, 1 minced garlic clove, and 1 teaspoon dried oregano for 6 to 9 minutes, or until the beef is browned. Add 4 ounces canned no-salt-added diced tomatoes, drained, or ½ cup fresh chopped tomatoes, 1 cup fresh or frozen broccoli florets, and the rice and cook until the broccoli is tender. Serve hot.
Total: 445 calories, 3 grams saturated fat, 8 grams fiber, 109 mg magnesium

WHOLE WHEAT PASTA WITH VEGGIES AND GARLIC STEAK

Prepare 1 cup cooked amount whole wheat pasta according to package directions. Drain and toss with ½ teaspoon olive oil, 1 tablespoon slivered fresh basil or 1½ teaspoons dried, and 2 tablespoons sunflower seed kernels. Coat a skillet with cooking spray and heat over medium-high heat. Cook 1 minced garlic clove, ½ cup chopped onion, and 1 cup sliced zucchini for 3 to 4 minutes, stirring often. Add 3 ounces extra-lean round steak sliced into thin strips, sprinkle with black pepper, and cook for 3 minutes, or until no longer pink. Serve over the pasta.
Total: 457 calories, 2 grams saturated fat, 8 grams fiber, 153 mg magnesium

BAHN MI

Heat 2 teaspoons canola oil in a small skillet over medium heat. Cook 3 ounces thinly sliced pork tenderloin for 3 minutes. In a small bowl, toss together ¼ cup shredded red cabbage, ¼ cup shredded green cabbage, 1 minced garlic clove, ¼ cup grated carrots, 2 tablespoons slivered almonds, 2 tablespoons chopped red onion, 1 tablespoon light mayonnaise, a few shakes of black pepper, and 2 teaspoons lime juice. Fold everything into a whole wheat wrap (about 100 calories and 5 grams fiber, such as Flat Out).

Total: 446 calories, 3 grams saturated fat, 12 grams fiber, 51 mg magnesium

ARTICHOKE PIZZA

Preheat the oven to 400°F. Place an 8" whole wheat pita on a baking sheet. Drizzle with 1 teaspoon olive oil, then top with 1 tablespoon chopped red onion; ⅓ cup artichoke hearts packed in water, drained; ½ cup baby spinach leaves; 3 ounces chopped roasted chicken breast; and ½ ounce shredded 75% reduced-fat Cheddar cheese. Bake for 6 to 8 minutes. Serve with a side of 1 cup sliced strawberries topped with 2 tablespoons low-fat vanilla yogurt. The pizza may be made ahead; heat in the microwave oven or eat chilled.

Total: 448 calories, 3 grams saturated fat, 14 grams fiber, 123 mg magnesium

MAPLE WALNUT QUINOA WITH ROASTED CHICKEN

Prepare ¾ cup cooked amount quinoa according to package directions. Toss with 1 teaspoon olive oil, 3 ounces diced roasted chicken breast, 1 tablespoon light maple syrup, 1 tablespoon walnuts, and ½ cup raspberries.

Total: 451 calories, 2 grams saturated fat, 8 grams fiber, 139 mg magnesium

CHICKEN AMANDINE AND LEMON PEAS

Heat 2 teaspoons olive oil in a skillet over medium heat. In a plastic bag, combine 1 tablespoon dried bread crumbs and 1 tablespoon slivered almonds. Shake one 4-ounce chicken breast in the mixture. Cook the chicken for 4 to 5 minutes on each side. In a microwave-safe bowl, combine 1 cup fresh or frozen peas with 1 teaspoon olive oil, 1½ tablespoons lemon juice, 1 minced garlic clove, and 1 or 2 shakes of onion powder. Cook in a microwave oven on high heat for 1 minute to 1 minute 15 seconds, or until the peas are cooked.

Total: 459 calories, 3 grams saturated fat, 10 grams fiber, 118 mg magnesium

Fish and Seafood Dishes

SALMON AND MANGO BERRY CHUTNEY

Combine 1 cup chopped mango and ¼ cup raspberries with 2 teaspoons chopped red onion, ½ teaspoon brown sugar, 1 shake of ground red pepper, and 3 shakes of ground cinnamon. Drain 5 ounces canned salmon and toss with the mixture. Serve with 2 slices multigrain cracker (with about 90 calories and 4 grams fiber).

Total: 450 calories, 2 grams saturated fat, 9 grams fiber, 68 mg magnesium

TILAPIA AND BASIL RASPBERRY PASTA

Prepare 1 cup cooked amount whole wheat pasta. Toss with 2 tablespoons raspberry vinaigrette dressing (about 65 calories' worth), a handful of fresh basil torn into small pieces, and ½ cup raspberries. Serve with 4 ounces roasted tilapia drizzled with 1 teaspoon olive oil and the juice of 1 lemon.

Total: 460 calories, 3 grams saturated fat, 8 grams fiber, 99 mg magnesium

FISH PAUPIETTE, SWEET POTATO, AND SPINACH

Preheat the oven to 410°F. Place 1 large sweet potato on a piece of foil and pierce it once or twice with a fork. Bake for 30 minutes. Meanwhile, place one 4-ounce, thin fillet sea bass (or grouper, cod, or halibut) on a baking sheet coated with cooking spray. Top with 1 teaspoon Dijon mustard, 1 teaspoon olive oil, 1 tablespoon whole wheat bread crumbs, and 2 teaspoons fresh basil or 1 teaspoon dried. Roll the fish and place it seam side down on a baking sheet. After the sweet potato has baked for 30 minutes, reduce the heat to 350°F, and bake both the fish and the potato for 7 to 9 minutes, or until the fish flakes with a fork. Serve the fish with half the sweet potato (save the rest for another meal, such as the Pecan Oatmeal on page 206), sprinkled with cinnamon and topped with 1 tablespoon trans-free spread. Serve with 1 cup spinach, from frozen, heated in a microwave oven and drizzled with 2 teaspoons olive oil and 2 shakes of ground red pepper, if desired.

Total: 449 calories, 4 grams saturated fat, 8 grams fiber, 233 mg magnesium

SNACKS

It's hard to go for hours without a meal, which is why we encourage snacking! It's a great way to keep your metabolism revved and reduce your overall calorie consumption. Sweet or savory, your snack cravings are covered here. Add two snacks to your daily diet—when you eat them is up to you. If you eat breakfast early, you may need a little something to tide you over until lunch. Almost everyone will need or want a snack between lunch and dinner. Or you can save one of your snacks and have a sweet treat for dessert. All of the snack ideas here have about 200 calories and at least 2 grams of fiber.

On the Sweet Side

RASPBERRY PANCAKES

Reheat the pancake from the Raspberry Pancakes breakfast (page 206), spread with 1 tablespoon all-fruit raspberry jam and topped with ½ cup raspberries.

Total: 204 calories, 1 gram saturated fat, 4 grams fiber

HOT COCOA AND CRUNCH

Mix 1 cup fat-free milk or plain soy milk with 2 teaspoons cocoa powder and 1 teaspoon sugar. Heat in a microwave oven on high for about 40 seconds (or serve chilled). Serve with 1 whole wheat cracker spread with 1 teaspoon peanut butter and topped with 1 teaspoon dried blueberries or 2 teaspoons raisins or dried cranberries.

Total: 195 calories, 1 gram saturated fat, 4 grams fiber

SORBET BERRY BOWL OR SMOOTHIE

Place ½ cup fat-free raspberry sorbet in a serving dish and top with ¼ cup each sliced strawberries, raspberries, and blackberries. Sprinkle with 1 tablespoon walnuts. If you prefer, toss all the ingredients into a blender and enjoy as a smoothie.

Total: 210 calories, 1 gram saturated fat, 7 grams fiber

STRAWBERRY YOGURT WITH CHOCOLATE-COVERED RAISINS

Combine ¾ cup fat-free plain yogurt with 1 cup sliced strawberries and 1 tablespoon chocolate-covered raisins.

Total: 194 calories, 2 grams saturated fat, 3 grams fiber

FRUITY BEAN YOGURT

Top ½ cup fat-free plain yogurt with 2 tablespoons dried blueberries or 3 tablespoons dried cranberries or raisins and 1 tablespoon jelly beans.

Total: 196 calories, 1 gram saturated fat, 2 grams fiber

BANANA SPLIT

Top 1 small banana with 2 tablespoons fat-free plain yogurt and 1 tablespoon each peanuts and chocolate chips.

Total: 208 calories, 3 grams saturated fat, 4 grams fiber

APRICOT COTTAGE CHEESE

Combine ⅔ cup fat-free cottage cheese with 1 or 2 drops of vanilla extract, 2 teaspoons all-fruit apricot preserves, and 3 sliced fresh apricots.

Total: 191 calories, 0 grams saturated fat, 2 grams fiber

PEACH SMOOTHIE

In a blender, combine 1 cup unsweetened frozen (or sliced fresh) peaches, 2 teaspoons honey, ½ cup fat-free plain yogurt, and 1 or 2 drops of vanilla extract.

Total: 207 calories, 0 grams saturated fat, 5 grams fiber

YOGURT WITH BANANA AND M&M'S MINIS

Have one 6-ounce fat-free Greek yogurt with half of a small banana, sliced; ½ cup sliced strawberries; and 1 tablespoon M&M's Minis.

Total: 190 calories, 2 grams saturated fat, 3 grams fiber

LÄRABAR ENERGY BAR

Have one of the following Lärabars: Chocolate Chip Brownie, Carrot Cake, Peanut Butter and Jelly, Cherry Pie, or Apple Pie.

Total: 190–210 calories, 0.5–2 grams saturated fat, 4–5 grams fiber

On the Salty/Savory Side

CUCUMBER SLIDERS

Top each of 3 whole wheat crackers (100 calories total) with 2 slices cucumber, ⅓ ounce reduced-fat Cheddar cheese, and a small dollop of Dijon mustard.

Total: 206 calories, 2 grams saturated fat, 6 grams fiber

CRACKERS WITH WALNUT-DATE SALAD

Toss ¼ cup mixed baby greens with ½ teaspoon olive oil and a splash of balsamic vinegar. Top 2 multigrain crackers (about 90 calories and 4 grams fiber) with the salad mixture, 2 teaspoons walnuts, and 2 chopped dates.

Total: 211 calories, 1 gram saturated fat, 6 grams fiber

FLAXSEED CRACKERS AND HUMMUS

Dip 8 flaxseed crackers (120 calories and at least 4 grams fiber, such as Dr. Kracker Organic and Artisan-Baked Snackers) in 2 tablespoons hummus mixed with 1 tablespoon dried cranberries or raisins.

Total: 193 calories, 2 grams saturated fat, 5 grams fiber

FLAXSEED CRACKERS AND SPICY AVOCADO DIP

Dip 8 flaxseed crackers (120 calories and at least 4 grams fiber, such as Dr. Kracker Organic and Artisan-Baked Snackers) in 3 tablespoons avocado mashed with 1 teaspoon lemon juice, 1 teaspoon chopped chili pepper, and a pinch of ground red pepper.

Total: 196 calories, 3 grams saturated fat, 7 grams fiber

CHIPS AND SALSA

Dip 1 ounce unsalted baked tortilla chips (about 18 chips) in 5 tablespoons no-salt-added salsa. Serve with 1 ounce low-fat string cheese.

Total: 185 calories, 2 grams saturated fat, 2 grams fiber

CUCUMBER AND TAHINI

Slice one-half cucumber. Dip slices into 2 tablespoons tahini.

Total: 200 calories, 3 grams saturated fat, 2 grams fiber

Sweet and Salty

CELERY WITH PEANUTTY RICOTTA DIP

Cut celery ribs into four 6" pieces. Dip in ¼ cup fat-free ricotta cheese mixed with 1 tablespoon dried strawberries and 2 teaspoons peanut butter.

Total: 194 calories, 2 grams saturated fat, 4 grams fiber

POPCORN PARTY MIX

Combine 3 cups reduced-fat microwave popcorn with 1 tablespoon pecans and 1 tablespoon M&M's Minis.

Total: 204 calories, 3 grams saturated fat, 4 grams fiber

PRETZEL SNACK MIX

Combine 1 ounce whole wheat pretzels with 1 tablespoon raisins and 2 teaspoons mini chocolate chips.

Total: 183 calories, 2 grams saturated fat, 3 grams fiber

CASHEWS AND PEACHES

Have 2 tablespoons cashews and 2 small peaches or 2 peach halves canned in juice.

Total: 191 calories, 2 grams saturated fat, 2 grams fiber

ALMONDY APPLE

Slice 1 small apple in half and remove the seeds. Top each half with 1 teaspoon almond butter and 5 almonds.

Total: 192 calories, 1 gram saturated fat, 5 grams fiber

TRAIL MIX

Have 2 tablespoons each dried cranberries, raisins, and peanuts, mixed together.

Total: 210 calories, 2 grams saturated fat, 3 grams fiber

PUDDING AND PECANS

Have 1 fat-free pudding snack, chocolate-vanilla swirl or vanilla flavor, along with 2 tablespoons pecans.

Total: 194 calories, 1 gram saturated fat, 2 grams fiber

WALNUTS AND RAISINS

Mix 3 tablespoons walnuts and 2 tablespoons raisins.

Total: 197 calories, 2 grams saturated fat, 2 grams fiber

CRUNCHY COTTAGE CHEESE BOWL

Have ¾ cup fat-free cottage cheese mixed with ¼ cup cereal (100 calories and at least 6 grams fiber per 1-cup serving) and 1 tablespoon sunflower seed kernels.

Total: 204 calories, 1 gram saturated fat, 3 grams fiber

BISCOTTI AND ALMONDS

Have 1 biscotti (about 100 calories' worth) and 2 tablespoons almonds.

Total: 200 calories, 3 grams saturated fat, 2 grams fiber

OPTIONAL SNACKS

If you're a man or a woman taller than 5′8″, you may need just a little more food to keep you satisfied. Enter this optional third snack. Each of the following has about 300 calories and at least 2 grams of fiber.

On the Sweet Side

CHOCOLATE RASPBERRY WAFFLE

Toast a frozen waffle (about 90 calories and at least 1 gram fiber). Top with ½ cup fat-free raspberry sorbet, 2 teaspoons peanuts, and 1 tablespoon chocolate chips.

Total: 296 calories, 3 grams saturated fat, 5 grams fiber

WHITE CHOCOLATE, PECANS, AND PRETZELS

Have 1.5 ounces pretzels, any style, with 2 teaspoons white chocolate chips and 1½ tablespoons pecans.

Total: 281 calories, 3 grams saturated fat, 2 grams fiber

CREAM CHEESE CRACKERS WITH CINNAMON-SUGAR PEANUTS

Preheat the oven to 350°F. Place 2 tablespoons peanuts on a piece of foil and drizzle with 2 teaspoons agave nectar or honey. Mix ¼ teaspoon cinnamon and 1 teaspoon sugar and sprinkle on top. Bake for 6 to 8 minutes. Spread 1 tablespoon reduced-fat cream cheese on 2 whole wheat crackers (90 calories and at least 4 grams fiber) and top with the peanuts.

Total: 296 calories, 3 grams saturated fat, 7 grams fiber

On the Salty/Savory Side

SHARP CHEDDAR TORTILLAS

In a microwave-safe bowl, top 1 ounce baked tortilla chips (about 18 chips) with 2 tablespoons salsa, ¾ cup fat-free refried beans, 1 thinly sliced green onion, 1 ounce low-fat shredded sharp Cheddar cheese, and ½ finely chopped jalapeño chile pepper, if desired. Heat in a microwave oven on high for 45 to 60 seconds, or until the cheese is melted.

Total: 285 calories, 1 gram saturated fat, 6 grams fiber

GRAB-AND-GO CHEESE, CRACKERS, AND RAISINS

Have 1 stick reduced-fat string cheese, 20 wheat crackers (150 calories' worth), and ¼ cup raisins.

Total: 303 calories, 3 grams saturated fat, 3 grams fiber

POPCORN AND PARMESAN

Have 6 cups reduced-fat microwave popcorn, sprinkled lightly with water and tossed with 2 tablespoons Parmesan cheese and ⅛ teaspoon crab-boil seasoning.

Total: 297 calories, 2 grams saturated fat, 7 grams fiber

BUILD YOUR OWN MEAL

Sometimes the easiest way to eat is to throw together a few items from your fridge and pantry. That's why we created our Build Your Own Meal chart, which allows you to assemble a healthy, tasty meal in just minutes while still meeting the goals of the Turn Up Your Fat Burn eating plan.

The meals listed on the previous pages include a combination of lean protein, whole grains, vegetables or fruits, and healthy fats (and a significant amount of fiber—at least 8 grams total per meal and 2 grams per snack). To create a balanced meal like these on your own, include one food from each category below. Add low-fat dairy (which can substitute for some of your lean protein portion), low-calorie flavor kickers, and treats as part of your meal as desired. We've listed calorie counts and fiber amounts in parentheses as a guide, but because servings and preparations can differ among brands, refer to package labels when possible. You can also read the nutrition facts label or look up nutrition facts online at www.usda.gov (click on Foods and Nutrition and What's in the Foods You Eat). Use any of these options to create your perfect meal or snack. Just be sure that you're still including a magnesium-rich food at least once a day (see the Maximum Magnesium list on page 194 for ideas).

Lean Protein

1 ounce roasted chicken breast (47 calories, 0 g fiber)

1 ounce broiled beef tenderloin (65 calories, 0 g fiber)

1 ounce baked turkey breast (48 calories, 0 g fiber)

1 ounce 90% lean ground beef, cooked (61 calories, 0 g fiber)

1 ounce steamed scallops (30 calories, 0 g fiber)

1 ounce broiled pink salmon (42 calories, 0 g fiber)

1 large egg (72 calories, 0 g fiber)

1 large egg white or 2 tablespoons egg substitute (16 calories, 0 g fiber)

1 ounce tofu (22 calories, 0.5 g fiber)

¼ cup black beans, canned (55 calories, 4 g fiber)

¼ cup white beans, canned (75 calories, 3 g fiber)

¼ cup kidney beans, canned (54 calories, 3.5 g fiber)

¼ cup lentils, cooked from dry (55 calories, 4 g fiber)

Whole Grain

1 ounce whole wheat bread
(80 calories, 2 g fiber)

½ ounce whole wheat crackers
(45 calories, 2 g fiber)

¼ cup cooked wild rice
(42 calories, 0.5 g fiber)

¼ cup cooked brown rice
(55 calories, 1 g fiber)

¼ cup cooked whole wheat
pasta (43 calories, 1.5 g fiber)

¼ cup whole wheat couscous
(79 calories, 1 g fiber)

1 ounce baked potato
with skin (28 calories, 0.5 g fiber)

1 ounce baked sweet potato
with skin (25 calories, 1 g fiber)

Vegetables and Fruits

1 cup spinach leaves (6 calories,
0.5 g fiber)

1 cup shredded romaine
(10 calories, 1 g fiber)

1 cup mixed baby greens
(7 calories, 1 g fiber)

¼ cup chopped red bell pepper
(12 calories, 1 g fiber)

¼ cup chopped green bell pepper
(7 calories, 1 g fiber)

¼ cup broccoli (8 calories, 0.5 g fiber)

¼ cup green beans (9 calories,
1 g fiber)

¼ cup carrots (11 calories, 1 g fiber)

¼ cup chopped scallions
(8 calories, 0.5 g fiber)

¼ cup chopped onion (16 calories,
0.5 g fiber)

¼ cup grape tomatoes (13 calories,
0 g fiber)

1 medium apple (95 calories,
4.5 g fiber)

1 cup cubed cantaloupe
(54 calories, 1.5 g fiber)

1 medium orange (62 calories,
3 g fiber)

1 cup strawberries (46 calories,
3 g fiber)

1 cup blueberries (83 calories,
3.5 g fiber)

1 cup raspberries (64 calories,
8 g fiber)

Healthy Fat

1 teaspoon olive oil (40 calories,
0 g fiber)

1 teaspoon canola oil (40 calories,
0 g fiber)

1 teaspoon sesame oil
(40 calories, 0 g fiber)

1 teaspoon light mayonnaise
(16 calories, 0 g fiber)

1 tablespoon sliced avocado
(15 calories, 1 g fiber)

1 tablespoon whole almonds
(54 calories, 1 g fiber)

Healthy Fat *(cont.)*

1 tablespoon chopped walnuts (48 calories, 0.5 g fiber)

1 tablespoon sesame seeds (52 calories, 1 g fiber)

1 tablespoon sunflower seeds (54 calories, 1 g fiber)

1 tablespoon pumpkin seeds (47 calories, 0 g fiber)

1 tablespoon hummus (25 calories, 0.5 g fiber)

1 tablespoon tahini (89 calories, 0.5 g fiber)

Low-Fat Dairy

1 ounce reduced-fat Cheddar cheese (67 calories, 0 g fiber)

1 ounce fat-free ricotta cheese (14 calories, 0 g fiber)

1 cup fat-free milk (83 calories, 0 g fiber)

1 cup 1% milk (104 calories, 0 g fiber)

1 cup fat-free plain yogurt (137 calories, 0 g fiber)

1 cup fat-free fruit yogurt (233 calories, 0 g fiber)

Treats

1 tablespoon chocolate chips (52 calories, 0 g fiber)

¼ cup fat-free sorbet (60 calories, 0 g fiber)

1 ounce baked tortilla chips (110 calories, 0 g fiber)

1 ounce baked potato chips (133 calories, 0 g fiber)

1 ounce pretzels (113 calories, 0.5 g fiber)

1 cup 94% fat-free microwave popcorn (20 calories, 0.5 g fiber)

Low-Calorie Flavor Kickers

½ teaspoon ground cinnamon (3 calories, 0.5 g fiber)

1 teaspoon garlic (4 calories, 0 g fiber)

1 teaspoon chopped serrano chile pepper (0 calories, 0 g fiber)

1 teaspoon chopped jalapeño chile pepper (0 calories, 0 g fiber)

½ teaspoon red-pepper flakes (3 calories, 0 g fiber)

1 tablespoon balsamic vinegar (0 calories, 0 g fiber)

Here are some examples of how you can put these foods together into meals. You'll notice that these sample meals include a magnesium-rich food (*italics*).

LEAN PROTEIN	WHOLE GRAIN	VEGETABLES AND FRUITS	HEALTHY FAT	DAIRY/TREATS/KICKERS
1 cup *black beans* (220 calories, 16 g fiber)	1 ounce whole wheat bread (80 calories, 2 g fiber)	3 cups mixed baby greens (21 calories, 3 g fiber) 1 cup strawberries (46 calories, 3 g fiber)	2 tablespoons sliced avocado (30 calories, 2 g fiber) 1 teaspoon olive oil (40 calories, 0 g fiber)	1 tablespoon balsamic vinegar (0 calories, 0 g fiber)

Directions: Spread whole wheat bread with sliced avocado and toss mixed baby greens and black beans with olive oil and balsamic vinegar. Have strawberries on the side.
- Calories: 437 • Fiber: 26 g

3 ounces broiled beef tenderloin (195 calories, 0 g fiber)	½ cup cooked wild rice (84 calories, 1 g fiber)	1½ cups sliced carrots (66 calories, 6 g fiber)	2 tablespoons *pumpkin seeds* (94 calories, 0 g fiber) ½ teaspoon canola oil (20 calories, 0 g fiber)	

Directions: Toss rice with pumpkin seeds and canola oil and serve with beef and carrots.
- Calories: 459 • Fiber: 7 g

2 ounces roasted chicken breast (94 calories, 0 g fiber)	¾ cup cooked *brown rice* (165 calories, 3 g fiber)	½ cup scallions (16 calories, 1 g fiber) 1 cup broccoli florets (32 calories, 2 g fiber)	1 teaspoon sesame oil (40 calories, 0 g fiber)	1 cup 1% milk (104 calories, 0 g fiber)

Directions: Stir-fry rice with the chicken, scallions, broccoli, and sesame oil. Have with milk.
- Calories: 451 • Fiber: 6 g

4 ounces baked turkey breast (192 calories, 0 g fiber)	½ cup cooked whole wheat couscous (158 calories, 2 g fiber)	4 cups *spinach leaves* (24 calories, 2 g fiber) ½ cup grape tomatoes, halved (26 calories, 0 g fiber)	1 teaspoon olive oil (40 calories, 0 g fiber)	

Directions: Toss spinach and tomatoes with olive oil and serve with turkey and couscous.
- Calories: 440 • Fiber: 4 g

4 ounces steamed *scallops* (120 calories, 0 g fiber)	¾ cup whole wheat spaghetti, cooked (129 calories, 4.5 g fiber)	1½ cups green beans (54 calories, 6 g fiber)	1 teaspoon garlic (4 calories, 0 g fiber) 2 teaspoons sesame oil (80 calories, 0 g fiber)	¼ cup fat-free sorbet (60 calories, 0 g fiber)

Directions: Toss scallops, garlic, spaghetti, and green beans with sesame oil. Have with sorbet.
- Calories: 447 • Fiber: 10.5 g

OUT AND ABOUT

We know you're busy and that sometimes the easiest way to eat is to stop at the drive-thru or sit down in a restaurant. In the real world, you eat out. That's why we put together this handy Out and About list with meal and snack choices available at some of the country's most popular fast-food and dine-in restaurants. If you don't see what you like on this list, check a chain restaurant's Web site. It's worth taking a moment to look up some of your favorite items and see how many calories and how much fat and fiber they contain.

When dining out, keep in mind the nutrition guidelines of the plan. Shoot for at least 8 grams of fiber at all meals and 2 grams in your snacks. In order to keep your saturated fat at 10 percent or fewer of daily calories, track your total daily of saturated fat grams. Keep the total at 16 or fewer grams per day if you're following 1,600 calories (19 grams max if you're following 1,900 calories). A good guideline is to limit your saturated fat to 4 grams per meal and 2 grams per snack, although you can vary the number per meal as long as you stay within your daily total.

On-the-Go Breakfasts

STARBUCKS

One Huevos Rancheros Wrap: 330 calories, 5 grams saturated fat, 8 grams fiber

Brewed (drip) coffee with 1 ounce (2 tablespoons) fat-free milk and 1 packet sugar: 37 calories

Total: 367 calories, 5 grams saturated fat*, 8 grams fiber

*Cut 1 gram saturated fat from elsewhere in your day.

McDONALD'S

Fruit'n Yogurt Parfait: 160 calories, 1 gram saturated fat, 1 gram fiber

Mix in your own bag of 1 cup of high-fiber cereal, such as Kashi Good Friends (170 calories, 12 grams fiber).

Total: 330 calories, 1 gram saturated fat, 13 grams fiber

SUBWAY

Subway Western Egg and Cheese Muffin Melt: 180 calories, 2 grams saturated fat, 6 grams fiber

Take along 1 large apple: 115 calories, 5 grams fiber.

Total: 295 calories, 2 grams saturated fat, 11 grams fiber

Subway Steak, Egg and Cheese Muffin Melt: 190 calories, 2.5 grams saturated fat, 6 grams fiber

Take along 1 large orange: 70 calories, 4 grams fiber.

Total: 260 calories, 2.5 grams saturated fat, 10 grams fiber

DENNY'S

Hearty Wheat Pancakes (2 pancakes): 310 calories, 0 grams saturated fat, 8 grams fiber

Top with ¼ serving (about 1 ounce) seasonal fruit: 18 calories.

Total: 328 calories, 0 grams saturated fat, 8 grams fiber

From the Sides menu, order 1 serving (4 ounces) egg whites (scrambled without oil), 1 toasted English muffin with no margarine (have half), spread with 1 tablespoon jam, plus 1 serving banana and 1 serving grapes.

Total: 316 calories, 0 grams saturated fat, 8 grams fiber

On-the-Go Lunch or Dinner

McDONALD'S

Hamburger: 250 calories, 3.5 grams saturated fat, 2 grams fiber

Premium Southwest Salad without Chicken: 140 calories, 2 grams saturated fat, 6 grams fiber

Newman's Own Low Fat Balsamic Vinaigrette or Newman's Own Low Fat Family Recipe Italian Dressing: 40–60 calories, 0 grams saturated fat, 0 grams fiber

Total: 430–450 calories, 5.5 grams saturated fat*, 8 grams fiber

*Cut 1 gram saturated fat from elsewhere in your day.

Strawberry Banana Smoothie, medium: 260 calories, 0 grams saturated fat, 3 grams fiber

Premium Southwest Salad without Chicken: 140 calories, 2 grams saturated fat, 6 grams fiber

Newman's Own Low Fat Balsamic Vinaigrette or Newman's Own Low Fat Family Recipe Italian Dressing: 40–60 calories, 0 grams saturated fat, 0 grams fiber

Total: 440–460 calories, 2 grams saturated fat, 9 grams fiber

---

BURGER KING

BK Veggie Burger: 410 calories, 2.5 grams saturated fat, 7 grams fiber

Side Salad: 40 calories, 1 gram saturated fat, 1 gram fiber

Ken's Fat Free Ranch Dressing, half packet: 30 calories, 0 grams saturated fat, 0 grams fiber

Total: 480 calories, 3.5 grams saturated fat, 8 grams fiber

APPLEBEE'S

Weight Watchers Paradise Chicken Salad: 340 calories, 1 gram saturated fat, 6 grams fiber

Seasonal Vegetables: 40–60 calories, 0 grams saturated fat, 2–3 grams fiber

Fresh Fruit, Side: 70 calories, 0 grams saturated fat, 1 grams fiber

Total: 450–470 calories, 1 gram saturated fat, 9–10 grams fiber

---

"Having a set plan got me started."

When she was a middle-school principal and district administrator, Patricia Rizzotto spent much of her time at work on her feet, walking between classrooms and meeting and checking up on the goings-on at her school. After retiring about 4 years ago, she noticed her weight gain—which had been gradually accumulating with each decade—suddenly seemed to accelerate. A broken foot that put her out of action for almost 5 months didn't help matters.

"Even my 89-year-old mother said she thought I'd put on weight," says Rizzotto, who decided it was time to take action. Although she'd lost weight successfully on other diets before, most of the time she gained it back—and then some. Having a structured exercise program to go with more thoughtful eating choices has made a difference. "I hadn't followed a prescribed weight-training and cardio plan before," she explains. "I usually just go in spurts." She says paying attention to how much she was eating and trying to get more fiber into her meals and snacks also made a big difference.

After 4 weeks on the plan, she dropped more than 4 pounds and reports that her back looks leaner, her pants feel looser, and most of her other clothes fit more comfortably. Even her mother has noticed. "She just told me I don't need to lose more weight—she thinks I look great now!"

WENDY'S

Large Chili: 330 calories, 4 grams saturated fat, 8 grams fiber

Garden Side Salad: 25 calories, 0 grams saturated fat, 2 grams fiber

Italian Vinaigrette Dressing: 70 calories, 1 gram saturated fat, 0 grams fiber

Total: 425 calories, 5 grams saturated fat*, 10 grams fiber

*Cut 1 gram saturated fat from elsewhere in your day.

Sour Cream and Chives Baked Potato: 320 calories, 2 grams saturated fat, 7 grams fiber

Garden Side Salad: 25 calories, 0 grams saturated fat, 2 grams fiber

Light Classic Ranch, half packet: 25 calories, 0.5 gram saturated fat, 0 grams fiber

Mandarin Orange Cup: 90 calories, 0 grams saturated fat, 1 gram fiber

Total: 460 calories, 4.5 grams saturated fat*, 10 grams fiber

*Cut 1 gram saturated fat from elsewhere in your day.

TACO BELL

Fresco Bean Burrito: 340 calories, 2.5 grams saturated fat, 11 grams fiber

Mexican Rice: 130 calories, 0 grams saturated fat, 1 gram fiber

Total: 470 calories, 2.5 grams saturated fat, 12 grams fiber

Tostada: 250 calories, 3.5 grams saturated fat, 10 grams fiber

Pintos 'n Cheese: 170 calories, 2.5 grams saturated fat, 9 grams fiber

Total: 420 calories, 6 grams saturated fat*, 19 grams fiber

*Cut 1 gram saturated fat from elsewhere in your day.

Fresco Crunchy Taco: 150 calories, 2.5 grams saturated fat, 3 grams fiber

Pintos 'n Cheese: 170 calories, 2.5 grams saturated fat, 9 grams fiber

Mexican Rice: 130 calories, 0 grams saturated fat, 1 gram fiber

Total: 450 calories, 5 grams saturated fat*, 13 grams fiber

*Cut 1 gram saturated fat from elsewhere in your day.

DUNKIN DONUTS

Egg White Veggie Flatbread: 330 calories, 5 grams saturated fat, 4 grams fiber

Garden Salad: 180 calories, 3 grams saturated fat, 4 grams fiber (removing as much cheese as possible reduces saturated fat to 0 grams and calories to 120)

Total: 450 calories, 5 grams saturated fat, 8 grams fiber

Skip the Salt

Most Americans consume twice the amount of sodium they should each day. The recommended guideline is just 2,300 milligrams of sodium, or the equivalent of about 1 teaspoon of salt, a day. About 80 percent of the sodium we eat each day isn't from the salt shaker; processed and packaged foods are loaded with it to preserve the food and add flavor.[18] That's especially true of low-fat foods, to which sodium is added to balance taste and texture.

Too much sodium is bad for your body—it significantly elevates your blood pressure and increases your risk of heart attack or stroke. Sodium can also make you feel bloated by increasing water retention (one more reason to drink lots of water, which will push out some of that extra sodium).

Here are some ways to limit the amount of sodium in your diet.

O Always check the sodium content of condiments, canned soup, and other prepared foods.

O Watch out for otherwise healthy choices that are sky-high in sodium. A fast-food chicken salad, for example, may have more than a third of your daily recommended intake, even without the dressing. Many frozen foods are also very high in sodium, so read labels before you buy. Look for products with no more than 150 milligrams of sodium per serving.

O Cut back on highly salted foods such as chips, packaged rice mixes, and nuts. If you're eating nuts, you can still have the salted kind—1 ounce has only about 80 to 120 milligrams sodium. Just don't mindlessly empty the entire bowl.

O Choose frozen vegetables over canned ones, which are typically very high in sodium.

O Rinse canned beans before cooking and you'll cut their sodium level by one-third.

O Skip the salt shaker at the dinner table or when you're cooking and sub in herbs and spices. You'll get a blast of flavor plus a dose of healthy phytonutrients.

Some of our favorite ways to season without salt:

The dish: beef
The spice: bay leaf, onion powder, sage, thyme, nutmeg

The dish: chicken
The spice: rosemary, tarragon, ginger, oregano

The dish: fish
The spice: dill, dry mustard, paprika, lemon juice

The dish: tomatoes/tomato sauce
The spice: bay leaf, basil, oregano

The dish: potatoes
The spice: dill, garlic, paprika, parsley

The dish: green beans, mixed baby greens, or spinach
The spice: tarragon, thyme, marjoram

CHILI'S

GG Asian Salad with dressing: 410 calories, 3 grams saturated fat, 8 grams fiber

Side order of Guacamole: 45 calories, 0 grams saturated fat, 2 grams fiber

Total: 455 calories, 3 grams saturated fat, 10 grams fiber

Black Bean Patty without bun: 200 calories, 0 grams saturated fat, 7 grams fiber

Side order of Guacamole: 45 calories, 0 grams saturated fat, 2 grams fiber

Side of Cinnamon Apples: 200 calories, 2 grams saturated fat, 7 grams fiber

Total: 445 calories, 2 grams saturated fat, 16 grams fiber

BOSTON MARKET

Roasted Turkey Breast, regular size (5 ounces): 180 calories, 1 gram saturated fat, 0 grams fiber

Fresh Steamed Vegetables: 60 calories, 3 grams fiber

Green Beans: 60 calories, 3 grams fiber

Garlic Dill New Potatoes: 140 calories, 1 grams saturated fat, 3 grams fiber

Total: 440 calories, 2 grams saturated fat, 9 grams fiber

On-the-Go Snacks

SUBWAY

Fruizle Express, Pineapple Delight with Banana: 160 calories, 0 grams saturated fat, 2 grams fiber

PANDA EXPRESS

Veggie Spring Roll (2 rolls): 160 calories, 1 gram saturated fat, 4 grams fiber

McDONALD'S

Small order French Fries: 230 calories, 1.5 grams saturated fat, 3 grams fiber

KFC

Side order of Potato Salad: 200 calories, 2 grams saturated fat, 3 grams fiber

Side order of Cole Slaw: 180 calories, 1.5 grams saturated fat, 2 grams fiber

TACO BELL

Fresco Grilled Steak Soft Taco or Fresco Ranchero Chicken Soft Taco: 160–170 calories, 1.5 grams saturated fat, 2 grams fiber

"I'm getting some of my speed back!"

A longtime runner, Cindy Wenrich knows how to train for a race—she even runs a half marathon every year. But when it came to losing some of the weight that seemed to be increasing each year, she needed help. "I've always done some form of cardio, but I never really understood how much cardio to do versus strength or something like yoga. I needed a plan."

A recent knee injury made coming back to running a little more difficult, and, after hitting nearly 160 pounds at 5'4", she blamed some of her injury on the extra weight. "Except when I was pregnant, I was never this heavy, and I could feel the extra stress on my knees."

Cindy liked the challenge the cardio intervals presented, especially while wearing a heart rate monitor. "I never did that kind of speedwork before. Looking at the heart rate monitor helps me to keep pushing so I don't fall back into my usual poky pace." But she credits the circuit training with creating some of the biggest changes. "I was using muscles I hadn't worked in a while, and I definitely started to see and feel a difference after a couple of weeks," she reports.

By the 4-week mark, Cindy had dropped nearly 6 pounds, including an inch off her waistline and ¾ inch off her hips. "My pants fit better; my jeans aren't so tight in the stomach, butt, and thighs; and overall, I feel my core is stronger and tighter."

That's also helped her get back to running. "I used to just concentrate on going out and doing 3 miles, but by doing the intervals, I've become a stronger, faster runner. It lets me do more in less time, so my workouts have become a lot more effective."

IN THE FROZEN AISLE

We've all been there—in a pinch for finding something healthy, filling, and fast, you reach into your freezer. Unfortunately, not all frozen meals are created equal. Many are loaded with sodium and have a surprisingly high fat content. As a rule, choose an entrée with about 450 calories, at least 8 grams of fiber, and no more than 4 grams of saturated fat.

It can be difficult to determine how much magnesium you're getting in your meal because product formulations change frequently, so make sure to eat at least one other magnesium-rich food in a different meal or snack that day. You may also need to supplement the meal with some fresh fruits or vegetables to boost your fiber intake.

Here is some of our favorite frozen fare.

AMY'S BLACK BEAN ENCHILADA WHOLE MEAL

1 gram saturated fat, 9 grams fiber

Total with ½ cup cooked brown rice: 439 calories, 1 gram saturated fat, 11 grams fiber

---

AMY'S BAKED ZITI BOWL

390 calories, 2 grams saturated fat, 6 grams fiber

Total with 1 cup blueberries: 452 calories, 2 grams saturated fat, 9 grams fiber

---

HEALTHY CHOICE ALL NATURAL ASIAN POTSTICKERS

380 calories, 1 gram saturated fat, 6 grams fiber

Total with 1½ cups strawberries: 449 calories, 1 gram saturated fat, 10 grams fiber

---

HEALTHY CHOICE ALL NATURAL PUMPKIN SQUASH RAVIOLI

300 calories, 2.5 grams saturated fat, 6 grams fiber

Total with 3 cups mixed baby greens with 2 teaspoons olive oil and a splash of balsamic vinegar: 421 calories, 3.8 grams saturated fat, 8 grams fiber

---

HEALTHY CHOICE CHICKEN BALSAMICO

350 calories, 1.5 grams saturated fat, 6 grams fiber

Total with 2 kiwifruit: 443 calories, 1.5 grams saturated fat, 11 grams fiber

KASHI SWEET & SOUR CHICKEN

320 calories, 0.5 gram saturated fat, 6 grams fiber

Total with 3 tablespoons mixed nuts: 447 calories, 2 grams saturated fat, 8 grams fiber

KASHI MAYAN HARVEST BAKE

340 calories, 1 gram saturated fat, 8 grams fiber

Total with 3 cups mixed baby greens with 2 teaspoons olive oil and a splash of balsamic vinegar: 461 calories, 2.3 grams saturated fat, 10 grams fiber

LEAN CUISINE JUMBO RIGATONI WITH MEATBALLS

400 calories, 3 grams saturated fat, 7 grams fiber

Total with 1 whole wheat cracker such as Wasa Multigrain: 445 calories, 3 grams saturated fat, 9 grams fiber

CHAPTER **12**

Recipes

Whether you're cooking for the whole family, looking to expand your healthy-food horizons, or just in the mood for something new, we've got almost 50 simple, delicious recipes to keep you satisfied. These meals require a little more work than the meal choices listed in Chapter 11, but they're still designed to be prepared relatively quickly and easily. (Most of the recipes can be made in 30 minutes or less.) All are packed with nutrition and flavor, without being high in calories or fat.

Start the day right with nine tasty breakfast choices, featuring everything from smoothies to cereal bars. All are about 300 calories or less and high in fiber. Next, mix and match from among the 20 hearty lunch or dinner options. We've also provided flavorful, effortless side dishes to round out each meal. Together, each meal comes in at about 450 calories and is high in fiber (at least 8 grams a serving). Many are also rich in magnesium, helping you reach your fill of this mighty mineral.

You'll also find 20 filling snack ideas, ranging from savory to sweet. All are 200 calories or less and contain at least 2 grams of fiber. By including two of these snacks in your eating plan, spaced throughout the day, you'll help keep your blood sugar levels steady and make sure your overall calories stay in check.

What Our Panelists Said

The members of the Turn Up Your Fat Burn panel didn't just test the exercises; most of them also took the time to make the recipes and meal ideas offered on these pages. Here's what they had to say about some of their favorites.

"I'm not a counter—I don't like to worry about how many calories or how much fat I'm eating. So I loved how easy it was to just try some of the recipes and ideas and use those as my guideline," says Leslie Kingston. "I was thrilled there were so many choices."

"I'm a big snacker, so I loved seeing so many snack options available to me," says Pam Garin, who counted the Pretzel Snack Mix on page 219 as one of her favorites.

"Portion control is really key for me, so following these meals and snacks was really important to keep me on track," notes Lisa Miller. "I discovered a lot of excellent new ideas that were so simple to prepare." One new food she's added to her diet: fish. "I used to eat a lot of chicken, and now I've discovered that making fish is so tasty and easy, not to mention healthy." (See three new fish recipes on pages 268–270.)

"I discovered how important it is to try something new," says Kathy Chartier. "I never really considered myself a whole grain person, but I discovered there were so many good whole wheat options out there that really taste good and are high in both fiber and magnesium." For more whole wheat pasta ideas, see Whole Wheat Pasta Salad with Peaches and Chickpeas (page 258) and Whole Wheat Pasta with Turkey Meatballs (page 264).

BREAKFASTS

Remember, your breakfasts should have about 300 calories and at least 8 grams of fiber. Many of these following recipes make multiple servings, so you can feed your family or save the rest for other mornings. The choices below cover both sweet and savory options and are perfect for mornings when you're in a rush and need something quick or for a more leisurely weekend morning meal. Remember, although you're not consuming as many calories at breakfast as in lunch or dinner, it's important to start your day with a morning meal in order to avoid overeating later in the day.

BBQ Cereal Mix

Makes 4 servings

1½ cups bran cereal

1½ cups toasted oat circle cereal, such as Cheerios

1 cup waffle-shaped rice cereal, such as Rice Chex

½ cup cashews

3 tablespoons golden or brown raisins

1 teaspoon brown sugar

⅛ teaspoon ground red pepper

⅛ teaspoon onion powder

⅛ teaspoon garlic powder

In a large bowl, mix the cereals, cashews, raisins, sugar, pepper, onion powder, and garlic powder. Divide into 4 servings. Store leftovers in an airtight container.

Per serving

Calories: 290
Protein: 9 grams
Carbohydrates: 52 grams
Fat: 9 grams
Saturated fat: 2 grams
Fiber: 12 grams
Sodium: 270 milligrams

Peanut Cereal Bars

Makes 8 servings

6 tablespoons brown sugar

4 tablespoons honey

½ cup peanut butter

5 cups cereal with about 120 calories and at least 6 grams fiber per cup, such as Kashi Good Friends

2 tablespoons peanuts

1 Heat a small saucepan over medium heat. Bring the sugar and honey to a boil, stirring occasionally. Remove from the heat and blend in the peanut butter. Stir in the cereal and peanuts.

2 Coat a 9" × 13" dish with cooking spray. Press the cereal mixture into the dish and allow to cool. When firm, cut into bars.

Per serving

Calories: 290
Protein: 8 grams
Carbohydrates: 50 grams
Fat: 10 grams
Saturated fat: 2 grams
Fiber: 8 grams
Sodium: 160 milligrams

Ginger Carrot Bars

Makes 8 servings

1 cup orange juice

⅔ cup rolled oats

1⅓ cups (8 ounces) pitted prunes

4 tablespoons water

1 cup whole wheat flour

1 cup cracked wheat bran

2 teaspoons baking powder

2 medium carrots, grated (about 1 cup)

⅓ cup light pancake syrup

½ cup egg substitute

2 tablespoons canola oil

2 tablespoons minced fresh ginger

2 teaspoons vanilla extract

½ cup dried sweetened cranberries

1 cup fresh or frozen raspberries, unsweetened

❶ Preheat the oven to 375°F. Coat a 9" × 13" baking dish with cooking spray.

❷ In a bowl, combine the orange juice and oats. Set aside to soften for 5 minutes.

❸ Combine the prunes and water in a food processor. Pulse until the prunes are finely chopped.

❹ In a large bowl, mix the flour, wheat bran, baking powder, carrots, prunes, syrup, egg substitute, oil, ginger, vanilla, and cranberries. Lightly stir in the reserved oats.

❺ Put the batter in the pan. Bake for 25 minutes.

❻ Top each serving with 2 tablespoons raspberries.

Per serving

Calories: 300
Protein: 8 grams
Carbohydrates: 59 grams
Fat: 5 grams
Saturated fat: 0 grams
Fiber: 9 grams
Sodium: 180 milligrams

Red Hot Eggs

Makes 4 servings

4 teaspoons olive oil

1 large onion, chopped

4 garlic cloves, minced

2 cups shredded romaine

3 chile peppers, chopped

¼ cup chopped cilantro

¼ teaspoon dried oregano

1½ cups egg substitute or 12 egg whites

4 whole wheat tortillas, each about 100 calories and with at least 5 grams fiber, such as Flat Out

⅔ cup fat-free sour cream

1 cup alfalfa sprouts

1 cup diced fresh tomatoes or no-salt-added canned stewed tomatoes, drained

1 Heat the oil in a skillet over medium-low heat. Cook the onion and garlic, stirring constantly, for 4 to 5 minutes, or until softened. Add the romaine, peppers, cilantro, and oregano. Cook about 3 minutes, or until the lettuce is limp. Remove to a bowl.

2 Coat the skillet with cooking spray and warm over low heat. Cook the egg substitute or egg whites for 3 to 5 minutes, stirring, until set.

3 Top each tortilla with one-quarter each of the eggs, chili mixture, sour cream, sprouts, and tomatoes.

Per serving

Calories: 300
Protein: 18 grams
Carbohydrates: 36 grams
Fat: 10 grams
Saturated fat: 2 grams
Fiber: 8 grams
Sodium: 460 milligrams

Italian Omelet

Makes 4 servings

1 cup egg substitute
  or 8 egg whites

2 eggs

5 teaspoons olive oil

¾ cup chopped green bell pepper

¾ cup chopped red bell pepper

½ cup oil-packed sun-dried
  tomatoes, drained and chopped

¼ cup reduced-fat shredded
  mozzarella cheese

12 whole wheat crackers,
   with 7 calories and 2 grams
   fiber per cracker, such as Wasa

1 In a bowl, whisk the egg substitute or egg whites and the eggs.

2 Heat the oil in a skillet over medium-low heat. Cook the eggs without stirring, for 4 to 6 minutes, until set on the bottom. Top with the peppers, tomatoes, and cheese and continue cooking until the eggs are completely set.

3 Fold the cooked eggs in half with a spatula and serve with crackers.

Per serving

Calories: 310
Protein: 17 grams
Carbohydrates: 38 grams
Fat: 12 grams
Saturated fat: 3 grams
Fiber: 8 grams
Sodium: 490 milligrams

Super Smoothie

Makes 1 serving

4 ounces silken tofu

¼ cup orange juice

1 tablespoon wheat germ

1 cup fat-free milk

1 cup fresh or frozen blueberries, unsweetened

½ cup fresh or frozen strawberries, unsweetened

¼ teaspoon vanilla extract

In a blender, combine the tofu, juice, wheat germ, milk, berries, and vanilla and blend. Serve immediately.

Per serving

Calories: 310
Protein: 17 grams
Carbohydrates: 54 grams
Fat: 4 grams
Saturated fat: 0 grams
Fiber: 11 grams
Sodium: 110 milligrams

Green Smoothie

Makes 1 serving

½ medium banana

1 kiwifruit

1¼ cups frozen chopped spinach

½ cup fat-free milk

1 teaspoon almond butter

1 teaspoon honey or agave nectar

In a blender, combine the banana, kiwifruit, spinach, milk, almond butter, and honey, and puree. Serve immediately.

Per serving

Calories: 310
Protein: 14 grams
Carbohydrates: 49 grams
Fat: 4 grams
Saturated fat: 0 grams
Fiber: 8 grams
Sodium: 223 milligrams

Banana Pancakes

Makes 4 servings

⅔ cup water

3½ tablespoons whole barley

1⅓ cups whole wheat flour

1½ teaspoons baking powder

½ cup fat-free milk

1 cup mashed banana

¼ cup egg substitute or 2 egg whites

2 tablespoons light maple syrup

2 tablespoons all-fruit preserves

1 cup orange segments

Per serving

Calories: 310
Protein: 10 grams
Carbohydrates: 68 grams
Fat: 2 grams
Saturated fat: 0 grams
Fiber: 9 grams
Sodium: 240 milligrams

1 In a small saucepan, bring the water to a boil. Add the barley and cook until all the water is absorbed and the barley is tender. (Or substitute ¾ cup cooked whole barley.)

2 In a medium bowl, combine the flour, baking powder, and cooked barley.

3 In a small bowl, combine the milk, banana, egg substitute or whites, and syrup. Stir into the dry ingredients.

4 Coat a skillet with cooking spray and heat over medium-high heat. Spoon in about ¼ cup of the batter for each pancake. Cook until bubbles form on the top, then flip and cook another minute. Transfer to a platter and keep warm. Repeat with the remaining batter.

5 Melt the preserves in the skillet, stirring. Add the orange segments and cook for 2 to 3 minutes, stirring occasionally. Divide the topping among the pancake servings.

Cinnamon French Toast

Makes 4 servings

½ cup fat-free half-and-half

½ cup egg substitute or 4 egg whites

⅛ teaspoon ground cinnamon

⅛ teaspoon nutmeg

8 slices whole wheat bread, about 80 calories and at least 2 grams fiber per slice

4 teaspoons canola oil, divided

6 peach halves canned in juice or water or 3 fresh peaches, sliced

1 cup fresh or frozen raspberries, unsweetened

1 In a bowl, combine the half-and-half, egg substitute or whites, cinnamon, and nutmeg. Dip the bread in the mixture to coat.

2 Heat 2 teaspoons of the oil in a large skillet over medium-high heat. Cook 4 slices of the bread for about 2½ minutes on each side, or until browned. Repeat with the remaining 2 teaspoons oil and 4 slices bread.

3 Serve topped with the peaches and raspberries.

Per serving

Calories: 310
Protein: 12 grams
Carbohydrates: 52 grams
Fat: 9 grams
Saturated fat: 1 gram
Fiber: 8 grams
Sodium: 420 milligrams

"I'm finally seeing a change for the better!"

Kathy Chartier says she never had a weight problem until she had two kids. Like many women, she found the baby weight never went away, and each year, the numbers on her scale began to gradually creep up. At 58 and with both of her kids out of college, she decided it was time to drop some of the 35 pounds she had put on since her twenties. Kathy began walking, doing yoga, and lifting weights on the resistance machines at her local Y, but she wasn't really seeing any results.

It wasn't until she started doing the Turn Up Your Fat Burn workout that the weight finally began to come off. After 1 month on the program, she lost 6 pounds and 5 inches, including 2 inches off her waist and 1¼ inches off her hips. "My pants are finally starting to feel looser, and my belly's not quite as flabby," she says. "And I can definitely see some definition in my arms!"

Kathy has noticed changes in her fitness level, as well. "I was walking my dog one afternoon, and a rainstorm started to roll in. We ended up running about ¼ mile home to beat the rain. I felt amazing that I could run that far without any problem!"

She also appreciated having a structured plan to follow over the 4 weeks she was on the panel. "On my second week doing the program, my husband had to go to the hospital, plus we were in the midst of planning a party for my son, which made my life chaotic," she says. "Despite all this, I was able to stay on track by combining my strength and cardio into one session, so the schedule was never too overwhelming."

And she's not stopping now. "I'm going to keep doing the intervals and circuits because it's definitely helping me get results," she adds. "I'm just getting started."

LUNCH/DINNER

T he lunches and dinners on the Turn Up Your Fat Burn eating plan are designed to be interchangeable. They're each about 450 calories, with at least 8 grams of fiber. Most have at least 20 percent of the daily value for magnesium (for that reason, we've provided the magnesium amount in the nutritional information for this section but not for breakfasts and snacks). You'll also see that many of the main dishes have suggested accompanying sides to make a complete meal; here you'll find nutritional information for both the main dish and the entire meal so that you can experiment with different sides if you prefer.

Basil, Bean, and Vegetable Stew

Makes 8 servings

3 tablespoons canola oil

2 medium onions, sliced

4 garlic cloves, minced

1 eggplant, cut into cubes

3 small zucchini, cut into slices

1 can (28 ounces) no-salt-added
stewed tomatoes

4 cups no-salt-added canned
cannellini beans

1 green bell pepper, cut into strips

1 red bell pepper, cut into strips

2 tablespoons chopped fresh basil

½ teaspoon ground black pepper

2 tablespoons chopped parsley

❶ Warm the oil in a large pot over medium-high heat for 1 minute. Cook the onions and garlic, stirring constantly, for 4 to 5 minutes.

❷ Add the eggplant, zucchini, tomatoes, beans, bell peppers, basil, and black pepper. Bring to a boil, then reduce the heat to low, cover, and cook, stirring occasionally, for 45 minutes, or until the vegetables are tender. Stir in the parsley before serving.

Per serving

Calories: 220
Protein: 9 grams
Carbohydrates: 31 grams
Fat: 7 grams
Saturated fat: 0 grams
Fiber: 10 grams
Sodium: 62 milligrams
Magnesium: 89 milligrams

Make It a Meal

Serve each bowl with 1 veggie burger, heated according to package directions, then spread with 5 teaspoons tahini.

Per meal: 450 calories, 3 grams saturated fat, 14 grams fiber

Red Lentil Soup with Lemon

Makes 8 servings

2 tablespoons olive oil

2 onions, thinly sliced

6 cups water

2 cups red lentils

1 teaspoon ground coriander

½ teaspoon salt

½ teaspoon ground black pepper

4 tablespoons lemon juice

2 cups parsley, chopped

1 Heat the oil in a large pot over medium heat. Cook the onion until translucent, about 5 minutes. Add the water, lentils, and coriander. Bring to a boil, reduce the heat, and simmer for 7 minutes, or until the lentils are soft but still hold their shape. Add the salt and pepper.

2 Just before serving, stir in the lemon juice and parsley.

Per serving
Calories: 220
Protein: 14 grams
Carbohydrates: 32 grams
Fat: 4.5 grams
Saturated fat: 0.5 grams
Fiber: 8 grams
Sodium: 164 milligrams
Magnesium: 13 milligrams

Make It a Meal
With each portion of soup, serve ½ cup quinoa cooked according to package directions, then tossed with 2 tablespoons chopped almonds, ½ teaspoon olive oil, and 1 teaspoon fresh basil.

Per meal: 450 calories, 2 grams saturated fat, 13 grams fiber

Mediterranean Beef Stew

Makes 8 servings

1½ pounds beef top round steak, cut into ¾"-long strips

4 garlic cloves, minced

3 cups reduced-fat, reduced-sodium beef broth

1 can (6 ounces) no-salt-added tomato paste

4 tablespoons red wine vinegar

1 tablespoon brown sugar

1 teaspoon ground cinnamon

½ teaspoon ground allspice

½ teaspoon ground cloves

¼ teaspoon ground black pepper

2 bay leaves

4 medium potatoes with skin, cut into ¾" cubes

3 medium onions, cut into thin wedges

1 pound mushrooms, sliced

2 green bell peppers, chopped

1 Coat the bottom of a large pot with cooking spray and warm it over medium-high heat. Cook the beef and garlic, stirring constantly, for 7 to 9 minutes.

2 Stir in the broth, tomato paste, vinegar, sugar, cinnamon, allspice, cloves, black pepper, and bay leaves. Add the potatoes, onions, and mushrooms. Bring to a boil, reduce the heat to low, cover and simmer for about 20 minutes.

3 Stir in the bell peppers. Cover and cook, stirring occasionally, for 20 minutes longer, or until the potatoes are tender. Discard the bay leaves.

Per serving

Calories: 210
Protein: 24 grams
Carbohydrates: 27 grams
Fat: 3 grams
Saturated fat: 1 gram
Fiber: 4 grams
Sodium: 239 milligrams
Magnesium: 22 milligrams

Make It a Meal
Serve each bowl of stew with 1 cup cooked edamame tossed with 1 teaspoon chopped parsley.

Per meal: 455 calories, 2 grams saturated fat, 12 grams fiber

Scallop and Potato Stew

Makes 8 servings

4 tablespoons canola oil

2 onions, chopped

4 garlic cloves, minced

4 strips turkey bacon, cut into ½" strips

6 cups water

2 cups white wine

½ teaspoon ground black pepper

1 teaspoon salt

½ teaspoon ground red pepper

4 teaspoons fresh oregano

4 teaspoons fresh thyme

4 teaspoons fresh rosemary

2 pounds small potatoes or 4 large potatoes, cut into ½" cubes

6 cups frozen corn

2 pounds fresh or frozen green beans

2 pounds sea scallops, halved

❶ Warm the oil in a skillet over medium heat. Cook the onion, garlic, and bacon, stirring often, for about 14 minutes.

❷ Add the water and wine, bring to a boil, then turn the heat to low and simmer for 10 minutes. Add the black pepper, salt, red pepper, oregano, thyme, rosemary, and potatoes. Cook for about 25 minutes, or until the potatoes are soft.

❸ Bring to a boil and add the corn, beans, and scallops. Reduce the heat to a simmer. Cover and cook for 4 minutes. Serve immediately.

Per serving

Calories: 450
Protein: 31 grams
Carbohydrates: 63 grams
Fat: 10 grams
Saturated fat: 1 gram
Fiber: 9 grams
Magnesium: 141 milligrams

Three Bean Salad

Makes 8 servings

¼ cup fruit or sherry vinegar

3 tablespoons white wine vinegar

3 tablespoons olive oil

2 garlic cloves, finely chopped

¼ teaspoon ground black pepper

3 cans (16 ounces each) no-salt-added red kidney beans, rinsed and drained

1 pound fresh or frozen sugar snap peas

1 pound fresh or frozen green beans

2 medium cucumbers with skin, diced

1 cup thinly sliced scallions

½ cup parsley, chopped

❶ In a large bowl, whisk the vinegars, oil, garlic, and pepper. Add the kidney beans and stir gently.

❷ Bring a large pot of water to a boil. Have a bowl of ice water nearby. Boil the sugar snap peas and green beans for 3 minutes. Drain and immediately chill in the ice water for 2 minutes. Drain. Add to the kidney bean mixture along with the cucumbers, scallions, and parsley and stir to combine.

Per serving

Calories: 240
Protein: 14 grams
Carbohydrates: 36 grams
Fat: 5 grams
Saturated fat: 1 gram
Fiber: 18 grams
Sodium: 79 milligrams
Magnesium: 71 milligrams

Make It a Meal
Serve each bowl with 2 ounces tempeh or 6 ounces tofu, cooked in 2 teaspoons sesame oil and sprinkled with 2 teaspoons sesame seeds.

Per meal: 450 calories, 4 grams saturated fat, 18 grams fiber

Tomato Cucumber Salad

Makes 8 servings

4 garlic cloves, minced

½ cup lemon juice

1 cup low-fat plain yogurt

¼ teaspoon ground black pepper

6 tablespoons Italian dressing (vinaigrette, not creamy)

½ cup fresh mint, chopped

½ cup parsley, chopped

2 medium cucumbers, chopped

6 medium tomatoes, chopped

2 slices whole wheat bread with crust, cut into ¾″ cubes

2 sprigs watercress, stems removed

2 red onions, thinly sliced

1 In a small bowl, combine the garlic, lemon juice, yogurt, pepper, dressing, mint, and parsley.

2 In a large serving bowl, combine the cucumbers, tomatoes, bread cubes, watercress, and onion. Pour the dressing over the salad and toss gently.

Per serving

Calories: 120
Protein: 5 grams
Carbohydrates: 21 grams
Fat: 3 grams
Saturated fat: 0 grams
Fiber: 4 grams
Sodium: 270 milligrams
Magnesium: 25 milligrams

Make It a Meal

Serve each portion of salad with ¾ cup cooked whole wheat penne pasta tossed with ½ cup no-salt-added chickpeas, 1 teaspoon olive oil, 2 teaspoons balsamic vinegar, and 1 teaspoon fresh basil or ½ teaspoon dried.

Per meal: 450 calories, 1 gram saturated fat, 17 grams fiber

Brown Rice and Cashew Salad

Makes 4 servings

½ cup brown rice

2 tablespoons unsalted cashews

1 onion, chopped

1 red bell pepper, chopped

1 tart apple such as Granny Smith, chopped

1 teaspoon fennel seed

½ cup apple juice

1 tablespoon honey

2 teaspoons canola oil

¼ teaspoon allspice

½ teaspoon cardamom

⅓ cup raisins

1 Cook the rice according to package directions. (Or substitute 1½ cups cooked brown rice.)

2 Preheat the oven to 350°F. Roast the cashews on a baking sheet for 4 to 6 minutes and set aside.

3 Coat a large skillet with cooking spray and warm over medium heat. Cook the onion and pepper, stirring often, for 5 minutes. Add the apple and cook, stirring, for 2 or 3 minutes, or until lightly browned. Stir in the fennel and cooked rice and heat until the rice is warm. Transfer to a serving bowl and top with the reserved cashews.

4 Whisk the apple juice, honey, oil, allspice, cardamom, and raisins and drizzle over the salad. Stir gently to mix.

Per serving

Calories: 230
Protein: 4 grams
Carbohydrates: 45 grams
Fat: 5 grams
Saturated fat: 1 gram
Fiber: 4 grams
Sodium: 5 milligrams
Magnesium: 60 milligrams

Make It a Meal

Serve each portion with 3 ounces broiled salmon and 15 medium asparagus spears drizzled with 1 tablespoon lemon juice.

Per meal: 460 calories, 3 grams saturated fat, 9 grams fiber

Whole Wheat Pasta Salad with Peaches and Chickpeas

Makes 4 servings

8 ounces whole wheat pasta

¼ cup rice wine vinegar

2 cups fresh or frozen sliced peaches, unsweetened

3 cups (18 ounces) low-sodium canned garbanzo beans, rinsed and drained

2 tablespoons chives, finely chopped

1 cup parsley, chopped

2 tablespoons olive oil

⅛ teaspoon salt

¼ teaspoon ground black pepper

8 cups baby spinach leaves

1 Cook the pasta according to package directions and drain.

2 In a large bowl, combine the vinegar, peaches, beans, chives, parsley, oil, salt, and pepper. Add the cooked pasta.

3 Serve chilled over the spinach.

Per serving

Calories: 440
Protein: 18 grams
Carbohydrates: 80 grams
Fat: 6 grams
Saturated fat: 1 gram
Fiber: 15 grams
Sodium: 210 milligrams
Magnesium: 203 milligrams

Cannellini, Corn, and Tomato Bread Salad

Makes 4 servings

½ cup fresh basil

⅓ cup walnuts

1 clove garlic

1 jalapeño chile pepper, seeded and stem removed

2 tablespoons white balsamic, white wine, or rice wine vinegar

3 tablespoons olive oil

⅛ teaspoon salt

¼ teaspoon ground black pepper

1 tablespoon water

3 cups (18 ounces) no-salt-added canned cannellini beans

4 slices whole wheat bread, cut in 1″ cubes

1 cup frozen white corn

3 cups diced tomatoes, fresh or no-salt-added canned

1 medium red or orange bell pepper, sliced

1 green or yellow bell pepper, sliced

1 In a food processor, combine the basil, walnuts, garlic, chile pepper, vinegar, oil, salt, black pepper, and water. Process for 1 minute and set aside.

2 In a large bowl, combine the beans, bread cubes, corn, tomatoes, and bell peppers. Add the reserved dressing and toss gently. Serve immediately.

Per serving

Calories: 450
Protein: 17 grams
Carbohydrates: 60 grams
Fat: 19 grams
Saturated fat: 2 grams
Fiber: 14 grams
Sodium: 310 milligrams
Magnesium: 137 milligrams

Asian Snow Pea and Asparagus Salad with Pork Tenderloin

Makes 4 servings

1 pound pork tenderloin, cut into 4 pieces

1 tablespoon olive oil

¼ teaspoon ground black pepper

1 cup quick-cooking brown rice

1 pound fresh asparagus, cut in 2" pieces

1 pound fresh snow peas

2 teaspoons canola oil

2 teaspoons sesame oil

3 tablespoons low-sodium soy sauce

3 tablespoons sesame seeds, toasted

½ cup sliced scallions

1 small jalapeño chile pepper, finely chopped

① Preheat the oven to 350°F. Coat a baking dish with cooking spray.

② Place the pork in the dish, drizzle with the olive oil, and sprinkle with the black pepper. Bake for 40 minutes.

③ Cook the rice according to package directions.

④ In a saucepan with enough water to cover the vegetables, boil the asparagus for 2 minutes, then add the snow peas and cook for 30 seconds more. Drain and chill under cold running water.

⑤ In a large bowl, combine the rice, 2 teaspoons canola oil, the sesame oil, and soy sauce. Add the snow peas, asparagus, and sesame seeds and stir to combine. Top the salad with the scallions and peppers.

⑥ Slice each portion of the pork and serve with one-fourth of the salad.

Per serving

Calories: 460
Protein: 35 grams
Carbohydrates: 51 grams
Fat: 13 grams
Saturated fat: 2 grams
Fiber: 9 grams
Sodium: 840 milligrams
Magnesium: 168 milligrams

Avocado and Turkey Melt

Makes 1 serving

1 slice whole wheat bread, toasted

3 ounces sliced turkey breast

1 slice tomato

½ ounce sliced reduced-fat
   Muenster cheese

¼ avocado, chopped

1 tablespoon salsa

1 Place the toast on a microwaveable serving plate. Arrange the turkey on the toast and top with the tomato and cheese. Heat in a microwave oven on high until the cheese is melted, about 1 minute.

2 Top with the avocado and salsa.

Per serving

Calories: 250
Protein: 25 grams
Carbohydrates: 18 grams
Fat: 9 grams
Saturated fat: 3 grams
Fiber: 4 grams
Sodium: 797 milligrams
Magnesium: 28 milligrams

Make It a Meal
Serve the sandwich with a side dish of 1 cup black beans mixed with the rest of the tomato, chopped; 2 teaspoons fresh basil; and 1 teaspoon olive oil.

Per meal: 450 calories, 3 grams saturated fat, 18 grams fiber

Sautéed Pepper and Chicken Sandwich

Makes 1 serving

¼ green bell pepper, sliced

¼ yellow bell pepper, sliced

3 slices red onion, each ¼" thick

3 black olives, sliced

¼ teaspoon dried oregano

1 teaspoon olive oil

2 teaspoons red wine vinegar

¼ teaspoon ground black pepper

1 (2-ounce) whole wheat roll

4 ounces roasted chicken breast

1. In a bowl, combine the bell peppers, onion, olives, oregano, oil, vinegar, and black pepper.

2. Coat a skillet with cooking spray and heat over medium heat. Add the pepper mixture and cook, stirring frequently, for 3 to 4 minutes.

3. Slice the roll and fill with the chicken and peppers.

Per serving

Calories: 330
Protein: 32 grams
Carbohydrates: 37 grams
Fat: 7 grams
Saturated fat: 2 grams
Fiber: 6 grams
Sodium: 513 milligrams
Magnesium: 85 milligrams

Make It a Meal

Serve each sandwich with ¾ cup cooked spinach (chopped, from frozen) dressed with ½ teaspoon olive oil and a sprinkle of ground red pepper.

Per meal: 440 calories, 2 grams saturated fat, 8 grams fiber

Stuffed Cheeseburgers

Makes 4 servings

1 cup whole mushrooms

1 medium onion

2 teaspoons canola oil

½ tomato

2 tablespoons parsley

1 tablespoon capers

2 tablespoons seasoned dry bread crumbs

¼ teaspoon ground black pepper

1 pound 93% lean ground beef

2 ounces 2% Cheddar cheese slices

1 Coat a grill rack with cooking spray. Preheat the grill to medium-hot.

2 In a food processor, finely chop the mushrooms and onion. Heat the oil in a large skillet over medium-high heat. Cook the mushrooms and onion, stirring frequently, for 4 to 5 minutes, or until tender. Transfer to a large bowl.

3 In a food processor, finely chop the tomato, parsley, and capers. Transfer to the bowl. Add the bread crumbs, pepper, and beef. Mix thoroughly and shape into 4 patties.

4 Grill for 5 minutes, then flip and top with the cheese. Cook for about 5 minutes more, or until a thermometer inserted in the center registers 160°F and the meat is no longer pink.

Make It a Meal

Serve each burger on a 1½-ounce whole wheat hamburger roll with at least 4 grams fiber, plus 1 table-spoon ketchup, if desired. On the side, have ¾ cup cooked spinach (chopped, from frozen) dressed with ½ teaspoon olive oil.

Per meal: 440 calories, 4 grams saturated fat, 8 grams fiber

Per serving

Calories: 230
Protein: 25 grams
Carbohydrates: 7 grams
Fat: 11 grams
Saturated fat: 4 grams
Fiber: 1 gram
Sodium: 176 milligrams
Magnesium: 9 milligrams

Whole Wheat Pasta with Turkey Meatballs

Makes 4 servings

3 cups fresh tomatoes or no-salt-added canned stewed tomatoes, coarsely chopped

½ teaspoon salt, divided

1½ teaspoons brown sugar, divided

2 cloves garlic

1 medium onion, chopped

9 ounces ground turkey breast

¼ teaspoon ground black pepper

1 teaspoon cinnamon

Pinch of allspice

½ cup raw pine nuts

1 lemon

8 ounces whole wheat pasta

4 tablespoons fat-free Greek yogurt

1 Preheat the oven to 375°F.

2 In a food processor, blend the tomatoes, ¼ teaspoon salt, sugar, and garlic.

3 In a large bowl, combine thoroughly the onion, turkey, remaining ¼ teaspoon salt, pepper, cinnamon, allspice, and pine nuts. Form into 1" meatballs. Coat a large, ovenproof, heavy-bottom skillet with cooking spray and heat over medium heat. Cook the meatballs for about 5 minutes, or until browned on all sides.

4 Pour the tomato mixture over the meatballs, squeeze the lemon over the mixture, and bake for 30 minutes.

5 Meanwhile, prepare the pasta according to package directions. Serve the meatballs over the pasta, topping each serving with 1 tablespoon of yogurt.

Make It a Meal
Serve each portion with a side of 3 cups mixed baby greens dressed with 2 teaspoons balsamic or red wine vinegar.

Per meal: 450 calories, 2 grams saturated fat, 9 grams fiber

Per serving
Calories: 440
Protein: 27 grams
Carbohydrates: 57 grams
Fat: 13 grams
Saturated fat: 2 grams
Fiber: 8 grams
Sodium: 362 milligrams
Magnesium: 156 milligrams

Chicken with Marinated Blueberries and Red Onions

Makes 4 servings

1 tablespoon olive oil

2 tablespoons red wine vinegar

½ teaspoon salt

½ teaspoon black pepper

½ cup finely sliced red onion

2 cups, fresh or frozen blueberries, unsweetened

1 pound rotisserie chicken, skin removed, cut into bite-size pieces

6 cups mixed baby greens or baby spinach

1 In a bowl, combine the oil, vinegar, salt, and pepper. Stir in the onion and berries.

2 In a large bowl, combine the chicken and greens. Dress with the blueberry mixture and serve.

Per serving

Calories: 280
Protein: 30 grams
Carbohydrates: 16 grams
Fat: 11 grams
Saturated fat: 3 grams
Fiber: 4 grams
Sodium: 770 milligrams
Magnesium: 26 milligrams

Make It a Meal

Serve each portion with a side of 1 cup cooked lima beans tossed with 1 teaspoon fresh dill or ½ teaspoon dried and ½ teaspoon olive oil.

Per meal: 460 calories, 3 grams saturated fat, 12 grams fiber

Dijon Grilled Chicken

Makes 4 servings

1 pound boneless, skinless chicken breasts

3 tablespoons Dijon mustard

¼ teaspoon black pepper

⅓ cup orange juice

2 teaspoons Worcestershire sauce

1 clove garlic, minced

1 Place the chicken in a shallow glass baking dish. Brush both sides with the mustard and sprinkle with the pepper.

2 In a small bowl, combine the orange juice, Worcestershire, and garlic. Pour half over the chicken and turn to coat. Cover and refrigerate for 30 minutes or overnight.

3 Coat a grill rack with cooking spray. Preheat the grill to medium-hot. Grill the chicken until cooked through, turning occasionally and brushing with remaining orange juice mixture, about 6 minutes on each side, or until a thermometer inserted in the thickest portion registers 160°F and the juices run clear.

Per serving

Calories: 150
Protein: 26 grams
Carbohydrates: 5 grams
Fat: 2 grams
Saturated fat: 1 gram
Fiber: 0 grams
Sodium: 430 milligrams
Magnesium: 35 milligrams

Make It a Meal

Serve each portion with a 1-ounce whole wheat roll, 1 serving Brown Rice and Cashew Salad (see page 257), and ½ cup sliced strawberries.

Per meal: 460 calories, 1 gram saturated fat, 9 grams fiber

Flank Steak with Edamame, Black Pepper, and Green Onions

Makes 4 servings

3 cups fresh or frozen edamame

12 ounces flank steak

2 tablespoons rice wine vinegar

4 teaspoons sesame oil

1 teaspoon minced fresh ginger

2 teaspoons minced fresh garlic

4 scallions, thinly sliced

¼ teaspoon salt

¼ teaspoon ground black pepper

1 Defrost the edamame at room temperature or under cold water. Pierce the steak several times with a fork, then cut in ¼" slices against the grain.

2 In a large bowl, combine the vinegar, oil, ginger, and garlic. Add the steak and marinate for 15 minutes at room temperature or up to 8 hours in the refrigerator, turning occasionally.

3 Coat a skillet with cooking spray and warm over medium heat. Cook the scallions, stirring constantly, for 1 minute. Add the beef with its marinade and cook, stirring constantly, for 4 minutes. Remove from the heat and add the edamame, salt, and pepper.

Per serving

Calories: 340
Protein: 30 grams
Carbohydrates: 15 grams
Fat: 16 grams
Saturated fat: 4 grams
Fiber: 6 grams
Sodium: 239 milligrams
Magnesium: 96 milligrams

Make It a Meal

Serve each portion with ½ cup cooked brown rice.

Per meal: 450 calories, 4 grams saturated fat, 8 grams fiber

Grilled Tuna with Fruit Kebabs

Makes 4 servings

1   can (8 ounces) pineapple chunks, packed in juice

⅓   cup orange juice

1   tablespoon low-sodium soy sauce

1   tablespoon sesame oil

2   teaspoons minced fresh ginger or ½ teaspoon ground

¼   teaspoon ground red pepper

1   clove garlic, minced

12   ounces tuna steaks, ¾" to 1" thick

1   navel orange, peeled and cut in 8 pieces

4   cherry tomatoes

1 Drain the pineapple, reserving the juice. In a large plastic bag, combine the pineapple juice, half the orange juice, the soy sauce, oil, ginger, pepper, and garlic. Add the tuna. Seal the bag and shake well to coat. Refrigerate for at least 30 minutes or overnight.

2 Coat a grill rack with cooking spray. Preheat the grill to medium-hot. Remove the fish from the marinade and grill, brushing with the marinade, about 5 minutes on each side, or until the fish is opaque.

3 Place the pineapple chunks, orange pieces, and tomatoes on skewers. Grill for 3 minutes, turn and brush with the remaining orange juice, and grill 3 minutes longer.

Per serving

Calories: 220
Protein: 21 grams
Carbohydrates: 17 grams
Fat: 8 grams
Saturated fat: 2 grams
Fiber: 2 grams
Sodium: 170 milligrams
Magnesium: 61 milligrams

Make It a Meal
Serve each portion with 1 serving Basil, Bean, and Vegetable Stew (see page 251).

Per meal: 440 calories, 2 grams saturated fat, 12 grams fiber

Cod in Cornmeal Crust with Chard

Makes 4 servings

½ cup cornmeal

1 teaspoon grated lemon peel

⅛ teaspoon salt

⅛ teaspoon ground black pepper

4 boneless cod fillet halves (4 ounces each) or rainbow trout, catfish, pollock, or orange roughy

2 tablespoons canola oil

8 cups Swiss chard, chopped

1 lemon

1 On a plate, combine the cornmeal, lemon peel, salt, and pepper. Moisten the fish with cold water and coat with the mix.

2 Heat the oil in a large skillet over medium heat. Cook the fish, skin side down, about 3 minutes, or until brown, then turn and cook about 2 minutes more, or until just opaque in the center. Remove from the skillet. Cook the chard, constantly turning, 2 to 3 minutes, or until wilted. Squeeze the lemon over the fish and chard.

Per serving

Calories: 230
Protein: 23 grams
Carbohydrates: 16 grams
Fat: 8 grams
Saturated fat: 1 gram
Fiber: 2 grams
Sodium: 290 milligrams
Magnesium: 115 milligrams

Make It a Meal

Serve each portion with ½ cup cooked whole wheat orzo tossed with 1 teaspoon chopped fresh parsley and 2 teaspoons olive oil.

Per meal: 460 calories, 2 grams saturated fat, 9 grams fiber

Broiled Rainbow Trout with Ginger

Makes 4 servings

1 pound rainbow trout fillets or cod, catfish, pollock, or orange roughy

4 teaspoons low-sodium soy sauce

¼ teaspoon ground black pepper

1 teaspoon minced fresh ginger or ½ teaspoon ground

2 tablespoons olive oil

¼ teaspoon paprika

❶ Preheat the broiler. Coat a shallow baking dish with cooking spray.

❷ Place the fish in the dish and sprinkle both sides with the soy sauce, pepper, and ginger. Drizzle with the oil and sprinkle with the paprika. Broil for 6 to 8 minutes, or until the fish flakes easily with a fork.

Per serving

Calories: 220
Protein: 24 grams
Carbohydrates: 1 gram
Fat: 13 grams
Saturated fat: 3 grams
Fiber: 0 grams
Sodium: 220 milligrams
Magnesium: 38 milligrams

Make It a Meal

Serve each portion with 1 portion Three Bean Salad (see page 255).

Per meal: 450 calories, 5 grams saturated fat, 9 grams fiber

"I'm satisfying my sweet tooth."

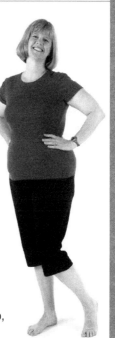

Although she was always tall and thin growing up, Audrey Stasak, 51, says putting on the freshman 10 in college was just the start of her gradual weight gain. Over the years, a job as a project manager meant more sitting than moving about, and her weight continued to creep up until she hit almost 210 pounds. "It's the heaviest I've ever been, and I realized I needed to do something," she says.

Working from home—and managing a serious sweet tooth—didn't help. "When I get done with a meeting, the refrigerator is always there," she says. Although she's followed traditional diets in the past, she hadn't put diet and exercise together. One of her favorite things about the plan is that it combines cardio, strength, and diet. "I liked the variety of the exercises and the challenge of changing the moves around each week."

At 5'11", Audrey added a third snack to help round out her diet, and she says a midday snack of some fruit and nuts or a fat-free ice cream bar were a great way to satisfy her sweet tooth. "Having just a little something goes a long way," she notes. Audrey also found herself drinking more water. "I bought an insulated glass to keep at my desk and sipped from it all day long," she says.

After a month, she'd lost about 5 pounds, including $\frac{1}{2}$ inch off her waist. "My clothes are all a little looser, and I can zip up some pants I couldn't even wear before!" She's also noticing more definition in her legs and arms and says her energy has doubled. "This has opened my eyes to a new way of exercising and eating. I'm looking forward to seeing more changes ahead."

SNACKS/DESSERTS

You'll eat two snacks a day—when is up to you. If you're an early breakfast eater, you may need a little something to tide you over until lunch. Almost everyone will want a snack between lunch and dinner. Or you can save one of your snacks and have a sweet treat for dessert. All of the snack ideas here have about 200 calories with at least 2 grams of fiber.

Vegetables with Almond Butter Dipping Sauce

Makes 1 serving

4 teaspoons almond butter

1 tablespoon orange juice

1 teaspoon rice vinegar

2 teaspoon peanuts

2 cups sliced cucumber, 1 cup sliced bell pepper, or ¾ cup baby carrots

In a bowl, combine the almond butter, juice, and vinegar and stir until smooth. Top with the peanuts. Dip the veggies in the sauce.

Per serving

Calories: 200
Protein: 8 grams
Carbohydrates: 15 grams
Fat: 14 grams
Saturated fat: 3 grams
Fiber: 3 grams
Sodium: 105 milligrams

Zesty Roasted Red Pepper Dip

Makes 1 serving

¼ cup finely chopped red bell pepper

1 teaspoon jalapeño chile pepper, finely chopped

4 tablespoons fat-free ricotta cheese

2 anchovy fillets canned in oil, drained, finely chopped

1 teaspoon lemon juice

1 teaspoon olive oil

2 whole wheat crackers (about 80 calories' worth)

In a bowl, combine the peppers, cheese, anchovies, lemon juice, and olive oil and mash with a fork. If you prefer a smoother texture, run the mixture through a food processor for 1 to 2 minutes. Chill until ready to eat. Dip the crackers in the mixture.

Per serving

Calories: 200
Protein: 10 grams
Carbohydrates: 28 grams
Fat: 6 grams
Saturated fat: 1 gram
Fiber: 5 grams
Sodium: 460 milligrams

Jicama with Grapes, Ricotta, and Almond Butter

Makes 1 serving

6 grapes, halved

2 tablespoons fat-free ricotta cheese

½ teaspoon almond butter

1 small jicama, sliced

In a small bowl, mix the grapes, cheese, and almond butter. Dip the jicama into the mixture.

Per serving

Calories: 200
Protein: 6 grams
Carbohydrates: 41 grams
Fat: 2 grams
Saturated fat: 0 grams
Fiber: 18 grams
Sodium: 60 milligrams

Spinach Spread

Makes 1 serving

2 cups fresh spinach

1 cup nonfat plain Greek yogurt

⅛ teaspoon nutmeg

⅛ teaspoon cinnamon

1 thin slice red onion

2 medium carrots, cut into sticks

In a food processor, blend the spinach, yogurt, nutmeg, cinnamon, and onion. Process for 1 minute, or until smooth. Dip the carrots in the mixture.

Per serving

Calories: 190
Protein: 22 grams
Carbohydrates: 26 grams
Fat: 0 grams
Saturated fat: 0 grams
Fiber: 6 grams
Sodium: 240 milligrams

Salsa with Baked Tortilla Chips

Makes 4 servings

1 can (16 ounces) no-salt-added diced tomatoes

3 jalapeño chile peppers, finely chopped

1 medium onion, finely chopped

1 tablespoon minced garlic

1 tablespoon cumin

1 teaspoon hot-pepper sauce

¼ teaspoon salt

¼ teaspoon ground black pepper

3 ounces baked tortilla chips

4 pieces (1 ounce each) light string cheese

1 In a bowl, combine the tomatoes, chile peppers, onion, garlic, cumin, hot-pepper sauce, salt, and black pepper. Chill at least 1 hour.

2 For 1 snack portion, serve one-quarter of the salsa with ¾ ounce, or about 13, baked tortilla chips and 1 ounce of the cheese.

Per serving

Calories: 200
Protein: 12 grams
Carbohydrates: 28 grams
Fat: 4 grams
Saturated fat: 2 grams
Fiber: 2 grams
Sodium: 500 milligrams

Kale Chips

Makes 4 servings (1¼ cups each)

6 cups chopped kale

1½ tablespoons olive oil

½ teaspoon salt, preferably sea salt

8 tablespoons unsalted mixed nuts

1 Preheat the oven to 400°F.

2 Spread the kale over a baking sheet. Drizzle with the oil and sprinkle with the salt. Bake for 12 minutes.

3 Have 1 serving of the kale chips with 2 tablespoons of the nuts. The rest of the kale chips can be stored for up to 2 days in a glass or plastic jar with a tight-fitting lid.

Per serving

Calories: 200
Protein: 6 grams
Carbohydrates: 14 grams
Fat: 15 grams
Saturated fat: 2 grams
Fiber: 4 grams
Sodium: 336 milligrams

Italian Bagel

Makes 1 serving

1 small whole wheat or oat bran bagel, or ½ large (about 150 calories)

2 tablespoons pasta sauce

2 tablespoons reduced-fat shredded mozzarella cheese

1 Preheat the oven to 200°F.

2 Cut the bagel in half and top with the sauce and cheese. Place on foil or a baking sheet and bake until the cheese begins to melt.

Per serving

Calories: 200
Protein: 11 grams
Carbohydrates: 35 grams
Fat: 3 grams
Saturated fat: 2 grams
Fiber: 5 grams
Sodium: 460 milligrams

Savory Dip

Makes 1 serving

½ cup fat-free plain yogurt

½ teaspoon dried dill

2 teaspoons lime juice

⅛ teaspoon horseradish sauce

2 tablespoons chopped scallions

10 baby carrots

5 cherry tomatoes

2 whole wheat crackers
  (80 calories' worth)

In a bowl, combine the yogurt, dill, lime juice, horseradish sauce, and scallions. Dip the carrots, tomatoes, and crackers in the mixture.

Per serving

Calories: 190
Protein: 9 grams
Carbohydrates: 43 grams
Fat: 0 grams
Saturated fat: 0 grams
Fiber: 8 grams
Sodium: 250 milligrams

Tomato and Flatbread Triangles

Makes 1 serving

2 medium tomatoes, chopped

1 whole wheat tortilla, about 120 calories, such as Flat Out

1 teaspoon finely chopped cilantro

1 teaspoon olive oil

2 teaspoons balsamic or red wine vinegar

1 Preheat the oven to 350°F. Coat a baking sheet with cooking spray. Bake the tomatoes for 17 minutes.

2 Reduce the heat to 200°F. Bake the tortilla on the center rack for 5 minutes. Break or cut into 4 triangles.

3 Toss the tomatoes with the cilantro, oil, and vinegar. Scoop with the tortilla.

Per serving

Calories: 210
Protein: 9 grams
Carbohydrates: 43 grams
Fat: 6 grams
Saturated fat: 1 gram
Fiber: 6 grams
Sodium: 290 milligrams

Sun-Dried Tomato Spread

Makes 1 serving

2 tablespoons oil-packed sun-dried tomatoes, drained and chopped

½ cup fat-free plain yogurt

1 teaspoon chopped fresh basil

½ teaspoon olive oil

2 whole wheat crackers (80 calories' worth)

In a bowl, combine the tomatoes, yogurt, basil, and oil. Spread on crackers.

Per serving

Calories: 200
Protein: 8 grams
Carbohydrates: 33 grams
Fat: 7 grams
Saturated fat: 1 gram
Fiber: 5 grams
Sodium: 200 milligrams

Blueberry Peach Shake

Makes 1 serving

3 tablespoons orange juice

¼ cup fat-free vanilla or peach frozen yogurt

2 ounces silken tofu

1 fresh peach or ½ cup frozen, unsweetened peach slices

½ cup fresh or frozen blueberries, unsweetened

1 In a blender, combine the juice, frozen yogurt, tofu, peaches, and half of the blueberries. Puree until smooth.

2 Pour into a glass, top with the remaining berries, and eat with a spoon.

Per serving

Calories: 200
Protein: 7 grams
Carbohydrates: 43 grams
Fat: 3 grams
Saturated fat: 0 grams
Fiber: 5 grams
Sodium: 40 milligrams

Maple-Pecan Oatmeal

Makes 1 serving

½ cup dry oats

2 teaspoons light maple syrup

1 tablespoon pecans

Prepare the oatmeal according to package directions. Stir in the maple syrup and pecans.

Per serving

Calories: 210
Protein: 6 grams
Carbohydrates: 31 grams
Fat: 8 grams
Saturated fat: 1 gram
Fiber: 4 grams
Sodium: 25 milligrams

Roasted Apple

Makes 1 serving

1 medium apple, halved and cored

½ teaspoon olive oil

1 teaspoon brown sugar

⅛ teaspoon dried thyme

1 tablespoon chopped walnuts

2 teaspoons reduced-fat sour cream

1 Preheat the oven to 225°F. Coat a baking dish with cooking spray.

2 Place the apple halves in the dish. Drizzle with the oil and sprinkle with the sugar, thyme, and walnuts. Bake for 16 to 18 minutes. Top with the sour cream.

Per serving

Calories: 190
Protein: 2 grams
Carbohydrates: 31 grams
Fat: 8 grams
Saturated fat: 2 grams
Fiber: 5 grams
Sodium: 10 milligrams

Strawberry Yogurt Freeze

Makes 1 serving

6 ounces fat-free strawberry yogurt

½ cup sliced strawberries

1½ tablespoons chopped pecans

⅛ teaspoon grated orange zest (optional)

Freeze the yogurt for at least 2 hours or up to 1 month. Scoop into a bowl and top with the strawberries, pecans, and orange zest, if desired.

Per serving

Calories: 200
Protein: 8 grams
Carbohydrates: 26 grams
Fat: 8 grams
Saturated fat: 1 gram
Fiber: 3 grams
Sodium: 85 milligrams

Pear with Almond Cream

Makes 1 serving

2 tablespoons reduced-fat sour cream

1 teaspoon brown sugar

2 drops almond extract

1 medium pear, halved and cored

1 tablespoon almonds

Mix the sour cream, sugar, and almond extract. Top the pear with the almond cream and sprinkle with the almonds.

Per serving

Calories: 210
Protein: 5 grams
Carbohydrates: 36 grams
Fat: 7 grams
Saturated fat: 2 grams
Fiber: 7 grams
Sodium: 36 milligrams

Espresso Parfait

Makes 1 serving

½ teaspoon instant espresso powder

2 tablespoons boiling water

1 plain biscotti, broken into small pieces

¼ cup fat-free frozen vanilla yogurt

2 teaspoons chocolate chips

¼ cup frozen blackberries, unsweetened

1 In a mug, dissolve the espresso powder in the boiling water. Let cool.

2 In a tall glass, layer a third of the biscotti pieces, half of the frozen yogurt, half of the espresso, and 1 teaspoon of the chocolate chips. Repeat. Top with the remaining biscotti pieces.

Per serving

Calories: 200
Protein: 5 grams
Carbohydrates: 35 grams
Fat: 5 grams
Saturated fat: 3 grams
Fiber: 2 grams
Sodium: 105 milligrams

Cappuccino Freeze

Makes 1 serving

½ cup fat-free vanilla frozen yogurt

2 teaspoons instant espresso powder

3 tablespoons boiling water

¼ teaspoon cinnamon

1 tablespoon unsalted cashews

½ cup fresh or frozen blueberries, unsweetened

❶ Thaw the frozen yogurt for 5 to 7 minutes.

❷ In a bowl, combine the coffee and water and stir until dissolved. Slowly beat into the frozen yogurt. Spoon into a bowl and top with the cinnamon, cashews, and blueberries.

Per serving

Calories: 200
Protein: 6 grams
Carbohydrates: 34 grams
Fat: 4 grams
Saturated fat: 1 gram
Fiber: 2 grams
Sodium: 65 milligrams

Sweet Potato Chips
and Raisin Apple Dip

Makes 1 serving

⅓ cup fat-free plain yogurt

¾ teaspoon fresh ginger, grated

½ teaspoon honey

1 tablespoon raisins

3 tablespoons chopped apple with skin

¾ ounce sweet potato chips

In a small bowl, combine the yogurt, ginger, honey, raisins, and apple. Scoop up with the chips.

Per serving

Calories: 210
Protein: 5 grams
Carbohydrates: 38 grams
Fat: 5 grams
Saturated fat: 1 gram
Fiber: 2 grams
Sodium: 55 milligrams

Crunchy Pistachio Pie

Makes 8 servings

4 tablespoons peanut butter

3 tablespoons honey

2 cups puffed rice cereal

1 package (1.5 ounces) reduced-calorie instant chocolate pudding

2 cups fat-free milk

3 tablespoons pistachios

3 tablespoons chocolate chips

1 cup sliced strawberries

1 Coat an 8" pie plate with cooking spray.

2 In a saucepan over low heat, warm the peanut butter and honey until the peanut butter has melted. Remove from the heat. Stir in the cereal. Press onto the bottom and sides of the pie plate.

3 Make the pudding with the milk according to package directions. Immediately pour into the prepared pie crust. Mix in the pistachios and chocolate chips. Refrigerate for at least 1 hour. Top with the strawberries and serve.

Per serving

Calories: 190
Protein: 6 grams
Carbohydrates: 24 grams
Fat: 8 grams
Saturated fat: 3 grams
Fiber: 2 grams
Sodium: 110 milligrams

Walnut-Cranberry Biscotti

Makes 8 servings

6 tablespoons walnuts, chopped

½ cup whole wheat flour

½ cup all-purpose flour

½ cup sugar

¼ cup unsweetened cocoa powder

½ teaspoon baking powder

¼ teaspoon baking soda

¼ teaspoon salt

1 egg

1 egg white

1½ teaspoons vanilla extract

¼ cup semisweet chocolate chips

3 tablespoons dried cranberries

1 Preheat the oven to 400°F.

2 Spread the walnuts on a baking sheet or foil and bake for 5 minutes. Reduce the heat to 350°F.

3 In a large bowl, combine the flours, sugar, cocoa, baking powder, baking soda, and salt. In a medium bowl, whisk together the egg, egg white, and vanilla. Add to the flour mixture and stir until smooth. Stir in the walnuts, chocolate chips, and cranberries.

4 Coat a 9" × 9" baking pan with cooking spray. Press the dough into the pan. Bake for 25 minutes, or until firm. Cool before serving.

Per serving

Calories: 190
Protein: 5 grams
Carbohydrates: 32 grams
Fat: 6 grams
Saturated fat: 2 grams
Fiber: 3 grams
Sodium: 160 milligrams

Real-Life Success | CATHERINE SCHAPER, 40

"I have more energy for my twin girls"

Twenty-three weeks into her pregnancy, Catherine Schaper was put on bedrest, where she remained until her twin daughters were born by emergency C-section. At that point, even walking around was difficult for Catherine, who hadn't gotten out of bed in 2 months.

As preemies, her daughters remained in the hospital for several weeks, which meant a constant back-and-forth. Once at home, one of the twins was diagnosed with a digestive issue that required round-the-clock monitoring. Finally, things calmed down enough for Catherine to think about getting back into shape. Several diets yielded quick results but equally quick rebounds. She found it hard to make time to exercise, and she needed a plan.

Although Catherine had been a regular gym-goer in the past, she didn't really push herself when she started exercising again. That changed on the Turn Up Your Fat Burn program. "I liked being able to work harder," she says. "During some of the exercises, I thought I couldn't do one more rep, but I always managed to finish." She also noticed a difference in her cardiovascular fitness. "As my conditioning improved, I recovered much more quickly and it was easier to stay in the zones."

Tweaks in her diet have also made Catherine feel healthier. "I was constantly munching off my kids' plates, finishing their food. Now I pay more attention to what I'm eating." Within a month, she dropped more than 5 pounds and lost about 2 inches. She also feels less bloated. And best of all, she has more energy for herself—and her kids. "The girls are 4½ now, and they want to do everything!"

"I realize I need to do something occasionally that is just for me, not for my family," she adds. "Some of that can wait—it's important for me to exercise, eat right, and set a good example."

Now What?

Y
ou've made it through the month and are probably asking yourself, "What do I do next?" After 4 weeks of following the Turn Up Your Fat Burn program, you're likely to have seen positive results, both physically (your clothes are looser, the number on the scale is lower, you're less tired at the end of the day) and mentally (you're more energized, more confident, and happier about your health and appearance). Even if you've achieved just one of these accomplishments, consider this past month a great success.

Consider all you've gained: You've made a substantial effort to improve your health and well-being. You've improved your cardiovascular conditioning and boosted the level at which your body burns fat. You've strengthened all your major muscle groups, revved your metabolism, and boosted your endurance.

But don't think of the plan as coming to an end. We hope you'll consider this just the beginning.

A month is not a lot of time to invest in your health. While you've seen changes for the better, you'll see even more if you keep up your exercise and healthy eating plan. Physical activity is meant to be done almost every day, not just in fits and starts. Now that you're moving, there's no reason to lose your momentum or undermine the gains you've worked hard to achieve.

PLANNING YOUR WORKOUTS

This is a good time to reread the science behind the Turn Up Your Fat Burn plan (see Chapters 1 and 2) so you have a greater understanding of what you've achieved so far. Recalling how and why the program was designed will help you continue to make progress.

Next it's time to plan the type and amount of exercise that will work best for you going forward.

At a minimum

Now that your 4-week plan is over, you may be wondering just how much exercise you need to commit to doing each week. At a minimum for good health, the American College of Sports Medicine recommends healthy adults do 30 minutes a day of moderately intense cardio (60 to 75 percent of maximal effort) 5 days a week, or 20 minutes of vigorous cardio (more than 75 percent of your max) 3 days a week, or any combination of the two. In addition, do some resistance

How Often Should I Weigh Myself?

The fit of your clothes is often a better guide than the scale. A little more room in the waistline or around the hips will provide a lot more positive feedback than a number will.

For the first couple of weeks on the plan, try skipping the weigh-in. It's common to not drop a lot of weight initially, which can be discouraging if you judge yourself by the scale. After that, a weekly weigh-in can provide some objective feedback. Do it about the same day and time each week—for example, Mondays at 7:30 a.m. before eating breakfast.

Another measure of success is body-fat percentage. Most health clubs can measure it for you, and so can many community and medical centers. Get a baseline, then follow-up measurements every few months. A change in body composition (less fat, more lean muscle) is a surefire way to let you know that your program is a success!

training 2 or 3 days a week, with at least one set of 8 to 10 reps for each major muscle group.[19]

Another minimal approach is to accumulate 30 minutes of moderate physical activity (such as walking, gardening, cleaning, climbing stairs, or playing with your kids) on most days, whether that's all together, in two 15-minute bouts, or divided into three 10-minute sessions.

Revisiting Your VT1

All of the interval workouts over the past month should have boosted your VT1 level. You should be able to work out more intensely (and therefore burn more calories) while keeping fat as the primary fuel

Four Ways to Mix Things Up

If you want to branch off the structured 4-week plan but continue to do some interval workouts, there's no shortage of ways to stay fit. Keep yourself challenged and avoid falling into a workout rut by mixing up your routine.

○ **Change the length of the "work" interval:** To make your workout harder, stay in the high-intensity zone for a longer time (for example, 30 seconds or 1 extra minute for each interval). You can make it easier, of course, by shortening the work interval.

○ **Change the length of the recovery:** The less time your body has to recover, the harder

the challenge. If you took 4 minutes to recover between intervals, cut it down to 3. Caution: Try not to go below 1 minute of recovery; you need some rest, or it's not a true interval routine—it's an all-out higher-intensity effort!

○ **Add intervals:** Don't be afraid to go for more. Increase the number of intervals you're doing as time permits.

○ **Intensity:** Up the intensity within the interval, working at a higher level (perhaps an RPE of 8 or 9 on a scale of 1 to 10), making sure you give yourself time to recover before hitting it again.

source. For example, if you've increased your base pace on the tread-mill from 3.5 mph to 4.0 mph, you're now burning 25 percent more calories with each workout—most of it still from fat.

One way to determine whether you've boosted your VT1 levels is to retake the test described on page 86. Pick a day when you haven't already done a strength workout (since that can skew your results), and do the same type of exercise you did for the original test a month ago: walking or running outside or on a treadmill, or using a bike, elliptical trainer, or stairclimber. If you used a heart rate monitor for the first test, wear one again to compare the hard numbers. If you're judging by RPE and the talk test, look at the numbers on the machine when you hit that point of breathlessness. Ideally, you'll be working at a higher level of intensity with speed, resistance/incline, or both.

Repeat the VT1 test every 4 to 6 weeks. If you continue training at and above VT1, you should continue to see the number rise. For exam-ple, if your heart rate was 135 beats per minute 4 weeks ago when you reached VT1, it may now be 140 beats per minute. You can work at a higher intensity level using your new VT1 as a guide.

Continue to challenge yourself as you go forward. On a treadmill, if you were at VT1 at 4.0 mph and a 2 percent incline a month ago, try increasing the incline to 3 percent and/or boosting your speed to 4.5 mph. Remember to keep using your RPE and talk test as a guide to stay just above your VT1.

Your work intervals should still feel like a good effort (you can say at least a few words at a time without having to take a breath) but not an impossible one (gasping for air or unable to talk at all). However, as your VT1 rises, you may go faster or against more resistance, which ultimately burns more calories.

What if your VT1 numbers haven't changed? Don't worry too much. Four weeks isn't a long time to follow a training regimen. Try alternat-ing workouts from Week 3 (a 5-minute work interval followed by a 4-minute recovery interval) and Week 4 (pushing to VT2 with short bursts of high intensity). Also, you can try adding a few more intervals to each session. Take the VT1 test again in another month and see if you've made progress. If you still haven't seen results, be honest about the level at which you're working—are you really pushing yourself to the point where your speech has become challenging but not difficult? Is your effort about a 7 on a scale of 1 to 10? All of us progress at our own speeds, but you should see significant improvement after 8 to 12 weeks of training, if you haven't already at 4 weeks.

CARDIO: MOVING ON UP

We encourage you to continue some form of interval training once or twice a week, along with two or three sessions of steady-state cardio—evenly paced workouts you can continue for 30 to 45 minutes with some effort. Steady-state is great for keeping your heart and lungs healthy and boosting your overall weekly calorie burn. However, as you've seen, intervals will continually improve your fitness levels and allow you to get more out of your workouts in less time.

You can continue to do some of the interval workouts in the Turn Up Your Fat Burn plan, adding more "work/rest" combinations as time allows. Instead of the three work/rest combos listed in Weeks 1 to 3, you can do four, five, or more. You can also lengthen your warmups and cooldowns or lengthen the steady-state exercise at your VT1 level. See "Four Ways to Mix Things Up" (page 296) for some ways to change up your interval program. You can also shift the work-to-recovery ratio, so you're working at a higher intensity for an even longer period, compared with your recovery time (for example, 2:1, 3:1, or 4:1 work-to-recovery intervals).

Here are a few cardio workouts to try as you move forward.

Sample 1: Interval Combos

This workout adds intervals while using a 4:3 work/recovery ratio. The warmup and cooldown are longer.

MINUTES	EFFORT	TALK TEST	HEART RATE (OPTIONAL)	RPE
0–5	Light (warmup) to medium	Easy conversation	Below VT1	3–4
5–9	Medium-high	Challenging (short phrases)	10 beats above VT1	7
9–12	Medium	Easier (short sentences)	Just below VT1	5
12–16	Medium-high	Challenging (short phrases)	10 beats above VT1	7
16–19	Medium	Easier (short sentences)	Just below VT1	5
19–23	Medium-high	Challenging (short phrases)	10 beats above VT1	7
23–26	Medium	Easier (short sentences)	Just below VT1	5
26–30	Medium-high	Challenging (short phrases)	10 beats above VT1	7
30–33	Medium	Easier (short sentences)	Just below VT1	5
33–37	Medium-high	Challenging (short phrases)	10 beats above VT1	7
37–40	Medium	Easier (short sentences)	Just below VT1	5
40–45	Medium, moving to light (cooldown)	Easy (full conversation)	Below VT1	3–4

Sample 2: Steady/Speed Mix-Up

This workout combines 20 minutes of steady-paced (at VT1) training (broken into two 10-minute blocks) with four above-VT1 speed or intensity intervals to boost your overall fitness and challenge your heart and lungs.

MINUTES	EFFORT	TALK TEST	HEART RATE (OPTIONAL)	RPE
0–3	Light (warmup)	Easy conversation	Below VT1	3–4
3–13	Medium	Somewhat breathless	VT1	5
13–16	Medium-high	Challenging (short phrases)	10–15 beats above VT1	7–8
16–19	Medium	Somewhat breathless	VT1	5
19–22	Medium-high	Challenging (short phrases)	10–15 beats above VT1	7–8
22–25	Medium	Somewhat breathless	VT1	5
25–28	Medium-high	Challenging (short phrases)	10–15 beats above VT1	7–8
28–31	Medium	Somewhat breathless	VT1	5
31–34	Medium-High	Challenging (short phrases)	10–15 beats above VT1	7–8
34–44	Medium	Somewhat breathless	VT1	5
44–48	Light (cooldown)	Easy conversation	Below VT1	3–4

Sample 3: Pyramid

The pyramid workout gradually builds intensity until halfway, when you're close to reaching VT2. From that point, every few minutes will get a little easier, so hang in there! It's a fun way to challenge yourself and keep from getting bored.

MINUTES	EFFORT	TALK TEST	HEART RATE (OPTIONAL)	RPE
0–3	Light (warmup)	Easy conversation	Below VT1	3–4
3–6	Increase speed or resistance slightly	Easy to moderate	Below VT1	4
6–9	Increase speed or resistance slightly	A little more breathless	Just below VT1	5
9–12	Increase speed or resistance slightly	Somewhat breathless/ choppy	At VT1	5–6
12–15	Increase speed or resistance slightly	Somewhat challenging	Just above VT1	6
15–18	Increase speed or resistance slightly	Challenging (short phrases)	10 beats above VT1	7
18–21	Increase speed or resistance slightly	Very challenging	15–20 beats above VT1	8–9
21–24	Decrease speed or resistance slightly	Challenging (short phrases)	10 beats above VT1	7
24–27	Decrease speed or resistance slightly	Somewhat challenging	Just above VT1	6
27–30	Decrease speed or resistance slightly	Somewhat breathless/ choppy	At VT1	5–6
30–33	Decrease speed or resistance slightly	A little breathless	Just below VT1	5
33–36	Decrease speed or resistance slightly	Easy to moderate	Below VT1	4
36–40	Light (cooldown)	Easy conversation	Below VT1	3–4

Other cardio choices

There's a world of workouts beyond these interval routines. Any aerobic activity is going to burn calories (including calories from fat) and help keep you fit, so don't limit yourself to the workouts in this book. The key is to do something you like. At least once a week, do something that doesn't involve a watch or a set program—anything that's just plain fun.

Pedal to work or around the neighborhood. Play a round of 18 on the weekend (but skip the cart and walk the course; you'll burn about 25 percent more calories). Play a game of doubles or singles tennis (singles burns about 25 percent more calories). Go for a hike, take a long walk, dive into a pool, find a pickup game of basketball. You're limited only by your interest and imagination.

METABOLIC STRENGTH WORKOUTS

Over the past 4 weeks (5 if you did the on-board week), you've challenged your muscles every which way, from combos that worked your whole body to balancing and jumping drills that boosted your overall fitness. By now you've discovered that regular strength training not only improves your muscle tone but makes you significantly stronger. So don't stop now!

Sticking with the routine

On the 4-week Turn Up Your Fat Burn plan, we increased the difficulty of the workouts pretty quickly. If at any point you had to modify or take a step back, consider going back to that week's workout and trying it again for another week. After a month of training, you may now be able to do balancing or multimuscle drills that seemed too difficult before. If you don't have joint or back issues, try the plyometric (jumping) exercises to boost your heart rate and up the intensity.

If you like the plan and want to do it again, begin with the Week 1 workout, but increase the challenge for each routine. If last month you did two circuits per routine, see if you can do three. You can also increase your overall work by lifting heavier weights (5-pound dumbbells

How Many Calories Can I Burn?

Want to know the calorie pay-off of all this moving around? Here's how many calories a 150-pound person will burn doing a particular activity for 1 hour. Heavier people typically burn more calories, lighter ones burn fewer. For a personalized calorie count, check out the My Health Trackers tool at prevention.com.

FITNESS FUN

Bicycling (leisurely pace, 10–11.9 mph)	408
Bicycling (moderate pace, 12–13.9 mph)	544
Bicycling (vigorous pace, 14–15.9 mph)	680
Boot camp class	544
Dance class	326
Hiking	408
Running (12-minute mile)	544
Running (10-minute mile)	680
Running (9-minute mile)	748
Run/walk combo (jogging less than 10 minutes total)	408
Stationary bike (150 watts, moderate effort)	476
Stationary bike (200 watts, vigorous effort)	714
Swimming freestyle (light effort)	476
Swimming freestyle (moderate; about 50 yards per minute)	544
Walking (20-minute mile)	224
Walking (17-minute mile)	258
Walking (15-minute mile)	340
Water aerobics class	272

SPORTS

Basketball (shooting around)	408
Basketball (playing a game)	544
Cross-country skiing (moderate pace)	544
Downhill skiing (moderate pace)	408
Golf (riding in cart)	238
Golf (walking with clubs)	306
Ice-skating	476
In-line skating	816
Kayaking	340
Racquetball	476
Soccer	680
Softball	340
Tennis (doubles)	408
Tennis (singles)	544
Volleyball (beach or indoor)	544

Calorie counts are based on the Compendium of Physical Activities Tracking Guide.

instead of 3, or 10-pound ones instead of 8) or boosting the number of repetitions (for example, 12 reps instead of the given 10). Longer workouts will improve your results and keep your muscles challenged. Or try adding a third day of circuit training each week (just make sure you have a full day's rest between workouts).

You can continue this plan for as long as you like, changing the routines a little less frequently (perhaps every 2 to 3 weeks instead of every week) or just repeating the 4-week program from the beginning every month, tweaking the weights and reps so you don't plateau.

A new routine

After a while, even the most enthusiastic exercisers can get a little bored in the weight room. Doing the same routine again and again can lead to a plateau in your results and a burnout in your attitude. Luckily, there are plenty of ways to add variety. The more you challenge yourself and surprise your muscles by switching things around, the more you'll rev your metabolism.

Customizing your strength routine is like cooking a meal. Start with the ingredients: your exercises. Put together combinations that work well together and that you like. Add spice with balancing or jumping elements.

Keep the circuit-training approach, going from one move to the next with minimal rest, then repeating all the exercises at least one more time. By mixing and matching exercises and creating new combos, you'll work your muscles in a variety of ways.

Read through the exercises listed beginning on page 306. Choose the moves you want to do, including at least one exercise for each major muscle group (chest, arms, shoulders, back, legs, glutes, and core). Combine a couple of exercises to work several muscles simultaneously. Add a balancing or jumping element if you want. It may help to write down the exercises you plan to do, in the order you wish to do them, before you start your workout. From week to week, you can vary the weight and rep count, using lighter weights and more reps or heavier weights and fewer reps.

You can find descriptions of many of these moves in this book. In addition, many exercises are shown in complete detail on the Web site of the American Council on Exercise. Go to acefitness.org and click on "Exercise Library" under the "ACE Get Fit" tab.

You can also incorporate basic fitness tools like resistance bands and stability balls into your routine. Resistance bands or elastic tubing work the muscles against resistance in a variety of angles. The bands are inexpensive (you can find them at sporting goods stores and mass merchants). You can easily bring them with you when you travel, too.

Stability balls, also called exercise balls or Swiss balls, are a great way to work your abdominal and back muscles while improving your stability. The balls have been used for years by physical therapists and are now a fitness staple. They add an element of instability to any exercise because you have to work to keep the ball from moving underneath you. Try using the ball instead of a weight bench to add a new challenge to moves like chest presses, planks, and rows. Or use the ball to increase the intensity of abdominal moves like crunches, twists, and back extensions.

Stability balls are also inexpensive and found at sporting goods stores and mass merchants. Buy one that's right for your height. When you sit on the ball, your hips should be level or just slightly higher than your knees.

4'11"–5'4": 55 cm

5'5"–5'11": 65 cm

6'0"+: 75 cm

Exercises in this book

You'll find all of these exercises in the on-board program or the 4-week plan. Mix and match in all-new ways to customize your routine. The exercises are arranged by targeted body part, but many work on multiple areas at once. In some cases, there are a couple of versions of the same exercise, with different challenges. This roundup pulls together variations introduced in different weeks of the workout, so you can see the progression and pick and choose.

Focus: Upper Body

Back
   Bent-over row (upper back), page 65
   Swimmer (back), page 71

Biceps
   Biceps curl (biceps), page 107
   Balancing alternating biceps curl (biceps, core, glutes), page 141
   Biceps blaster (biceps), page 167
   Concentration biceps curl (biceps), page 168

Chest
   Pushup (chest, arms, abs), page 70
   Pushup with row (chest, triceps, core, upper back), page 121
   Decline pushup (chest, core), page 162
   Chest press (chest, triceps, shoulders), page 101
   Chest press/fly combo (chest), page 123
   Standing dumbbell fly (chest, core), page 163

Shoulders
   Seated overhead press (shoulders), page 69
   Standing shoulder press (shoulders), page 104
   Balancing shoulder press/triceps extension (shoulders, triceps, core, glutes), page 142

Variations

Try these simple variations that tweak the moves you've already done in the Turn Up Your Fat Burn workout plan. Challenge yourself and avoid boredom by incorporating some of these new moves into your ongoing routine.

Focus: Upper Body

Incline chest fly *(chest)*

How to: Do a chest fly, but use a bench that's inclined 30 to 45 degrees.

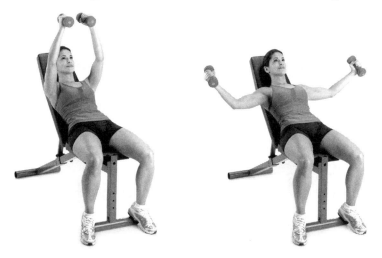

Stability ball press *(chest, triceps, abs)*

How to: Do a chest press, using a stability ball instead of a bench.

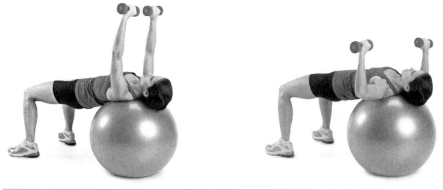

Stability ball fly *(chest, abs)*

How to: Do a chest fly, using a stability ball instead of a bench.

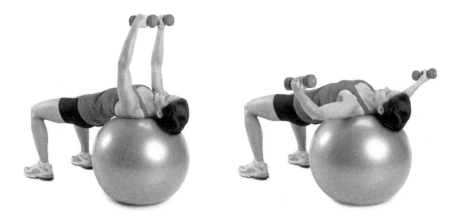

Incline pushup *(chest, shoulders, triceps)*

How to: Do a pushup with your hands on a bench and legs extended on the floor behind you.

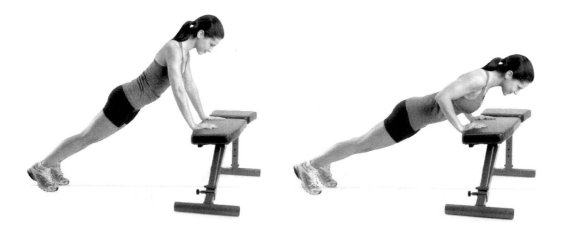

Ball pushup *(chest, shoulders, triceps)*

How to: Do a modified pushup with your hands on a stability ball, your knees on the floor.

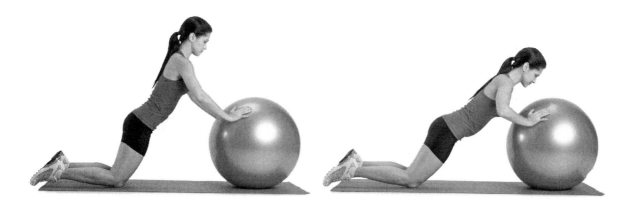

Pushup with single-leg raise *(chest, shoulders, triceps, glutes)*

How to: Do a pushup, but keep one leg lifted; switch legs halfway through the set.

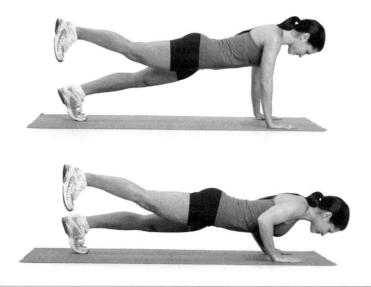

Front raise *(shoulders)*

How to: Raise the weights in front of you to chest height, your arms straight but not locked.

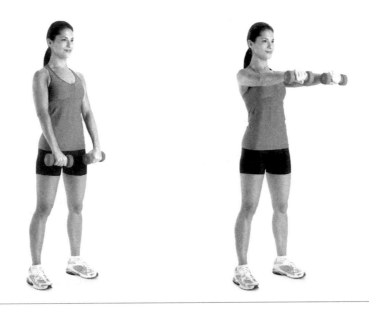

Hammer curl *(biceps)*

How to: Do a regular biceps curls with your palms facing each other, thumbs up.

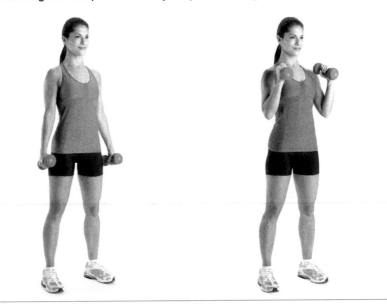

Focus: Lower Body

Ball squat *(glutes, quads)*

How to: Place the ball behind you against a wall and squat down, keeping your knees over your ankles.

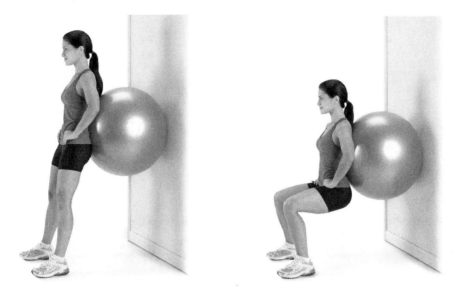

Single-leg bridge *(glutes, hamstrings)*

How to: Do a bridge, but extend and straighten one leg.

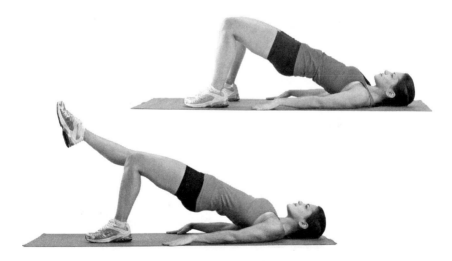

Bridge on ball *(hamstrings, glutes)*

How to: Place both feet on a stability ball instead of the floor and lift your hips.

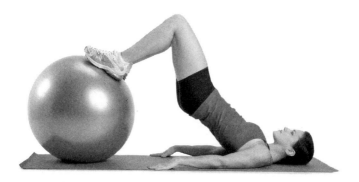

Ball curl *(hamstrings)*

How to: Place both feet on the ball, lift your hips, and curl the ball toward your body.

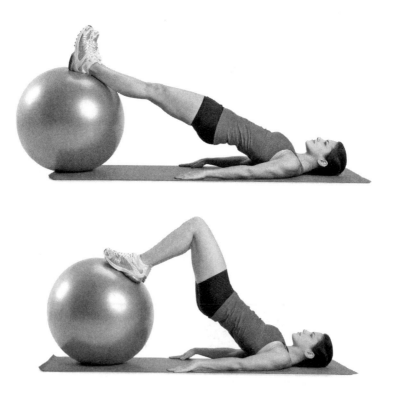

Mountain climber *(glutes, hamstrings, quads, abs)*

How to: Place your hands on the floor, your legs extended, and alternate bringing your legs toward your chest.

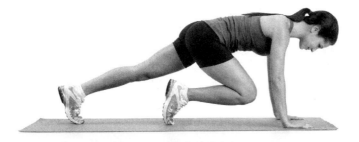

Focus: Core

Ball crunch *(abdominals)*

How to: Do crunches while sitting on a stability ball.

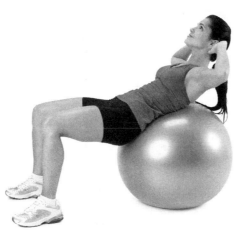

Stability ball knee tuck *(abdominals)*

How to: Lie on top of the ball and walk your hands out so you're in a pushup position, with your shins on the ball. Draw your knees toward your chest, then push the ball back to the starting position, keeping your torso stable.

Russian twist *(obliques)*

How to: Sit on the floor with your knees slightly bent and your heels on the floor, holding a weight or medicine ball in both hands. Lean back, keeping your abs tight. Rotate your torso as far as you can to the left, then go back to center and to the right.

Quadruped *(core, lower back)*

How to: Begin on all fours, your knees under your hips and your palms under your shoulders. Lift your right arm and left leg; hold for a moment, then bring your elbow to meet your knee under your chest. Do all the reps and repeat.

Build a Stronger Core

To get a lean, toned midsection, you'll need to work all of your core muscles, which include the following:

- **Rectus abdominus:** Also known as the "six-pack," this muscle group is usually only seen when body fat levels are low.

- **Internal/external obliques:** These muscles run down the sides of the abdomen, helping you rotate and bend at the sides. The internal obliques lie deeper within the body while the external obliques are more superficial (toward the surface).

- **Transverse abdominus:** Considered your body's natural girdle, this deep layer of muscles wraps around your middle, providing support to your spine.

- **Erector spinae:** Rounding out your core is the erector spinae group, which runs along the lower back and the spine.

If we can't see these muscles, why do we care about them? Working these muscles will not only help the ones you *can* see look even better, they make daily tasks (like bending and lifting) easier. Because the Turn Up Your Fat Burn plan incorporates so many different types of motion, you're already working them all.

Take it to the gym

Keep it fresh and work your muscles in a new way with these additional exercises that use equipment commonly found at fitness centers. For expert advice on how to do them, check out the detailed descriptions in the ACE Fitness exercise library at acefitness.org/exerciselibrary.

Focus: Upper Body

Chinup or assisted chinup *(biceps, upper back)*

Equipment: Pullup bar or assisted chinup machine

Seated row *(upper back, biceps)*

Equipment: Cable machine or resistance band

Standing row with machine or tubing

(biceps, upper and lower back, posterior shoulders, core)

Equipment: Cable machine or resistance band

Pullup or assisted pullup *(upper back)*

Equipment: Pullup bar or assisted pullup machine

Lat pulldown *(upper back)*

Equipment: Lat pulldown machine

Focus: Lower Body

Seated leg press *(quads, glutes)*

Equipment: Seated leg-press machine

Standing leg extension *(thighs, core)*

Equipment: Cable machine or resistance band

Standing hip adduction *(outer thighs, glutes, core)*

Equipment: Cable machine or resistance band

Standing hamstring curl *(hamstrings, core)*

Equipment: Cable machine or resistance band

Put it together

Create your own metabolic strength circuit: You can do any of the moves individually or combine them (as in the Turn Up Your Fat Burn plan) to work several muscles simultaneously. Vary the focus so you're not working the same muscle group too many times in a row. Always begin your workout with a brief warmup of dynamic stretches. Follow these simple guidelines when putting your metabolic circuit workout together.

○ **Work large before small.** Focus on larger muscle groups (chest, back, glutes, quads, hamstrings) before smaller muscles (triceps, biceps, shoulders, calves).

○ **Go up and down.** If you're focusing on one major muscle group at a time, alternate between upper- and lower-body moves (for example, a pushup followed by a squat, a row followed by a lunge). You're resting one muscle group while working the other. This also keeps blood pumping through your body (a process called peripheral heart action, or PHA), which will ultimately burn more calories.

○ **Give yourself a little time to recover.** Choose your priority for the workout. To make your circuit more aerobic, shorten the rest between each exercise (a minimum of 10 seconds, to set yourself up correctly). Rest longer and you may be able to lift a little more weight, which will help add muscle mass.

Sample Circuit 1: At home (no equipment)

1. Bodyweight squat (quads, glutes)
2. Pushup (chest, arms, abs)
3. Around-the-clock lunge (glutes, quads, outer thighs, inner thighs)
4. Plank (abs, lower back)
5. Plank combo (abs, obliques, hips, shoulders)
6. Step–up and hold (quads, glutes)
7. Triceps dip (triceps)

8. Bridge (hamstrings, glutes)

9. Crunch series (abs, obliques)

Sample Circuit 2: At home, with dumbbells, single-focus exercises

1. Chest press (chest, triceps, shoulders)

2. Romanian deadlift (hamstrings, glutes)

3. Seated overhead press (shoulders)

4. Side lunge (outer thighs, glutes)

5. Lateral raise (sides of shoulders)

6. Concentration biceps curl (biceps)

7. Plié squat (glutes, quads, outer thighs)

8. Overhead triceps extension (triceps)

9. Standing torso twist (obliques)

Sample Circuit 3 : At home, with dumbbells, combo exercises

1. Pushup with single-leg raise (chest, shoulders, triceps, glutes)

2. Single-leg deadlift with row (hamstrings, glutes, upper back)

3. Squat with shoulder press (quads, glutes, shoulders)

4. Lunge with triceps kickback (quads, glutes, triceps)

5. Plié squat with heel lift and biceps curl (outer thighs, quads, glutes, calves, biceps)

6. Curtsy lunge with lateral raise (shoulders, quads, outer thighs, glutes)

7. Wood chop (quads, glutes, obliques, shoulders)

8. Plank combo (abs, obliques)

Sample Circuit 4: Balancing and plyometric exercises

1. Jumping squat (glutes, quads, core)

2. Balancing alternating biceps curl (biceps, core, glutes)

3. Scissor lunge (quads, glutes, calves)

4. Balancing triceps extension (triceps, abs)

5. Mountain climber (glutes, hamstrings, quads, abs)

6. Single-leg squat (glutes, quads, core)

7. Balancing overhead press (shoulders, core)

8. Burpee (arms, chest, shoulders, legs, glutes)

9. Single-leg deadlift (hamstrings, glutes, core)

10. Side plank (obliques, hips)

Sample Circuit 5: Balls and bands

1. Stability ball press (chest)

2. Stability ball fly (chest)

3. Seated row with band (upper back, biceps)

4. Standing row with tubing (biceps, upper and lower back, shoulders, core)

5. Ball squat (quads, glutes)

6. Bridge on the ball (hamstrings, glutes)

Don't Just Live for the Weekend

For many of us, the weekend is a time to lean back and relax, which can also mean taking a couple of days off from watching what we eat. Be careful: A study of long-term dieters found that those who consumed about the same amount of calories on the weekend as during the week were 1.5 times more likely to keep off a weight gain of 5 pounds or more than those who dieted more strictly on weekdays but let loose on the weekend.[20]

7. Ball curl (hamstrings)
8. Ball crunch (abs)
9. Tabletop twist on ball (obliques, glutes)

Sample Circuit 6: At the gym

1. Stability ball press (chest, triceps, abs)
2. Pullup or assisted pullup (upper back)
3. Seated row (upper back, biceps)
4. Triceps dip (triceps)
5. Seated overhead press (shoulders)
6. Lat pulldown (upper back)
7. Seated leg press (quads, glutes)
8. Standing leg extension (thighs, core)
9. Standing hamstring curl (hamstrings, core)
10. Standing hip adduction (outer thighs, glutes, core)
11. Standing torso twist (obliques)
12. Bicycle (abs, obliques)

YOUR EATING PLAN

For the past few weeks, we've asked you to control portion sizes, include plenty of fiber, drink lots of water, snack a couple of times a day to keep yourself satisfied, choose magnesium-rich foods, eat whole grains, enjoy lots of fruits and vegetables, and choose healthy fats. These aren't short-term, fad-diet tips. They're part of following a well-balanced diet for the rest of your life.

But real life means you may have to face the occasional dietary challenges. One week might be particularly crowded with parties and get-togethers, so you'll need to be a little more vigilant about how much you're consuming in one sitting. Family gatherings and parties don't happen every day, though, so don't pass up your favorite foods every single time there's a celebration; give yourself permission to indulge once in a while. Other times you might find yourself so busy that you forget to eat. Don't worry about one bad meal or even one bad week. The important thing is to get back on the path you've started down.

By now, you know what works best for you. If you feel your eating is getting out of control, step back and remind yourself how to keep those calories in check. Starting a food journal again can be a good way to put meals and snacks under the microscope and show just how much you're eating and how often.

It's also important to plan ahead for both workouts and meals. Figuring out the logistics can keep your health habits on track. At least a day or two ahead, determine which workout you want to do and when, as well as what food you need to stock up on and when you're going to prepare it.

Lessons from the real biggest losers

Back in the very first chapter, we mentioned the National Weight Control Registry. If you really want to keep weight off over the long term, learn from the people tracked by that study. The registry, established in 1994 by researchers at Brown Medical School and the University of Colorado, is the largest investigation of long-term successful weight-loss maintenance. It tracks more than 5,000 individuals who have lost at least 30 pounds and kept it off for a year or longer. These real-world "biggest losers" have a number of things in common.[21]

○ **78 percent eat breakfast every day.** Starting the day off with a healthy meal helps keep you from overeating later in the day.

In It for Life

For the nearly two dozen men and women on the Turn Up Your Fat Burn test panel, exercise and eating right have become habits they plan on keeping up for the long haul. "When something feels good, you don't want to let it go," says Kimberly Hampsey. Here are a few of their favorite lasting benefits—beyond weight loss—after their 4 weeks on the program.

○ **More energy.** "There's nothing like working with young kids to realize how quickly you're getting out of shape," notes Hans Wagner, who works with preschool and elementary schoolchildren. "I can't believe how much more energy and endurance I have now that I've been working out consistently on the plan."

○ **Less stress.** "I have a natural inclination to be a little depressed, but doing this exercise program helped me manage my stress levels and kept me from feeling too blue," says Loretta Marsicano.

○ **Better organization.** "In the past, most of my workouts were on a whim—whatever I felt like doing that day," says Wendy Klemka. "Following this routine has kept me honest and more in line—so I know what I'm doing, and I get the payoff I'm looking for."

○ **Increased calorie burn.** "I've always exercised regularly, mostly walking, and I thought I usually went at a pretty good clip. But when I started to do the intervals, I realized I could take the intensity level up significantly—all the way into a jog rather than my usual power walk!" declares Anne Jenkins.

○ **Ready to take on the world!** "I feel fantastic after I do the workouts. My shirt is soaked, my heart rate is revved, and I feel a huge sense of satisfaction," says Michael Waverly. "It's rewarding to be able to work hard and get that extra boost in your day."

○ **75 percent weigh themselves at least once a week.** Because weight can fluctuate from day to day, stepping on the scale every morning or evening can be disconcerting. But weighing yourself once a week seems to offer enough of a check-in to keep you on track and help you become more aware of any significant fluctuations or trends.

○ **62 percent watch fewer than 10 hours of TV a week.** Sitting on the couch with the clicker can be dangerous in many ways. It's a pretty basic formula: The less active you are, the higher your chances of gaining significant weight. A recent study from Vanderbilt University of more than 30,000 women found that among white women, those who were the most sedentary were 4.5 times more likely to be severely obese. African-American women were 1.5 times more likely to fall into this group.[22] The Nurses' Health Study found that, even taking exercise into account, every additional 2 hours a day spent watching television increases the risk of obesity by 23 percent and the risk of diabetes by 14 percent.[23] Why is spending time with the small screen such a danger to your waistline? For one, if you're skipping a workout in favor of a date with *Dancing with the Stars,* you're missing an opportunity to burn off extra calories. Watching TV can also be a backdrop for mindless eating. Even a healthy snack can become dangerous when eaten in excess—if you're not paying attention, a handful of nuts can soon lead to the whole can. And the Nurses' Health Study found that the more TV women watch, the more they tend to eat high-fat, low-fiber, and high-calorie foods. (Guess all those fast-food commercials get through.)[24] That doesn't mean you can't tune in to your favorite reality show or settle down for the nightly news. Just make an effort to get up every few minutes. Use a commercial break to stretch, walk around the room, or just stand up and move. And make sure you incorporate walking breaks into the rest of your day. In the Nurses' study, researchers found that each hour spent walking briskly (not necessarily all at once) was associated with a 24 percent reduction in obesity and a 34 percent reduction in diabetes.[25]

- **90 percent exercise, on average, about 1 hour per day.** That means 9 out of every 10 people who have lost 30 pounds or more and kept if off include some form of regular exercise in their daily routine. You don't have to spend that hour in one single block. Try breaking it up into a few smaller workouts (a brisk 15-minute walk in the morning, another one at lunch, and a half-hour workout after dinner). If you make the workouts more vigorous (like many of the routines in the Turn Up Your Fat Burn plan), you can cut that time dramatically. The more exercise you do, the better you'll be at fighting off unwanted weight gain—especially when it comes to dangerous belly fat. A study from Duke University found that subjects who walked on a treadmill an average of 11 miles a week over 8 months were able to prevent an increase in visceral fat; those who logged an average of 17 miles a week actually lost 8 percent of deep belly fat on average. A sedentary group, on the other hand, gained 9 percent overall visceral fat in the same time frame.[26]

More ways to keep off the weight

- **Get a good night's sleep.** Numerous studies have shown that when people are better rested, they're less likely to gain weight. A Canadian study found that people who averaged 7 to 8 hours of sleep a night were 35 percent less likely to gain more than 10 pounds than those who snoozed 5 to 6 hours a night. The sleepy heads also had nearly 60 percent more fat around the middle.[27] Experts speculate that chronic sleep deprivation can alter the level of hormones affecting appetite and the way we process and store carbs. There's also a link between lack of sleep and increases in the stress hormone cortisol, which is associated with weight gain in general and belly fat in particular.

- **Stay in touch.** When you have followed a plan with specific day-to-day and week-to-week guidelines, it can sometimes be difficult to establish a routine on your own. Of course, you can always reboot and repeat the program from Week 1. But eventually, you'll need to come up with a regular routine. After the past few weeks, you have the basics down: Do some form of cardio (including intervals) at least 3 days a week and some form of strength training at least twice a week. And keep track of what you're eating. It can help to continue to write down your progress and even record it online. A Kaiser Permanente study found that individuals who checked into a Web site at least once a month to record their weight or food consumption over $2\frac{1}{2}$ years maintained an average of 9 pounds of their original 19-pound weight loss. Those who checked in regularly for only 14 months were able to maintain only 5 pounds of their weight loss.[28] Use the My Health Trackers tool on prevention.com to help you stay on top of your exercise and diet choices.

○ **Be as active as you can.** The more you move throughout the day, the better off you are, both for your health and your pant size. Walk the perimeter of the grocery store before you head toward the items you need. Move in place while you're on the phone. Park at the far end of the mall parking lot so you'll walk for a few minutes before you get to the stores. Stroll around the block at lunch and after dinner. Take the stairs instead of the elevator. (One study found that two additional minutes of climbing stairs a day, covering approximately three floors, can burn enough calories to eliminate the average American's annual weight gain of 1 to 2 pounds.) If possible, walk to do your errands instead of driving. Each hour behind the wheel has been associated with a 6 percent increase in obesity.[29] All of these little movements can lead to hundreds of extra calories burned by the end of the week.

○ **Keep making small changes.** You've done a lot over the past few weeks to get yourself healthier and in shape. So don't stop now! Research shows that people who make small, permanent changes in their food choices and/or physical activity each week lose significantly more belly fat and weight than those who simply diet or work out. That's because small changes lead to healthy behaviors that last. So to control the portion size and calorie content, try brown-bagging your lunch once a week instead of eating out (you'll save thousands of calories and hundreds of dollars a year!). Continue to eat more fruit and veggies so you're getting plenty of fiber along with important vitamins and minerals. Try brushing your teeth and flossing after dinner to take away the urge to snack on something sweet. All of these small changes can make a big difference in the long run. And they're likely to last.

In conclusion . . .

You hold in your hands a book that will serve as a roadmap to better health and wellness. But don't let the journey end here. You're well on your way, and it's just the beginning. Come back and revisit the information on these pages any time you need a little motivation, are looking for a new challenge, or just want a "reset" button. Your body is a wonderful machine, and if you treat it well with the right nutrition and exercise, it will reward you in kind with more energy, stamina, strength, and satisfaction. You'll burn fat more efficiently and keep your metabolism revved through the days and years ahead. And it will help you live a healthier, happier, fitter life. Enjoy it.

Journal

Research has proven that keeping a journal is one of the best ways to change your eating and exercise habits and lose weight for good. In one study of 1,600 people in four different U.S. cities, those who recorded their meals and activity levels 7 days a week lost twice as much weight over 6 months as their nonjournaling counterparts. That's because a journal keeps you honest by helping you account for your time. A reminder of that midnight snack or an empty exercise log can inspire you to do better next time, but it's also a record of your positive progress on your weight loss and fitness journey.

We have provided 1 week of blank journal pages that you can photocopy to help track yourself as you follow the plan. Before you get started, take some time to weigh and measure yourself—you can enter your results under the Starting Stats on page 330. We've provided room to record your weight, body circumference measurements, and even your bloodwork numbers (with the help of a doctor) as they are, at the beginning of the program. This way, as the weeks go by, you'll be able to see just how far you've come, stay on track, and meet your goals! On the following pages, you can record your starting VT1 threshold. You'll want to keep this important info handy while you're working out, and reassess every 4 weeks or so as you get more fit and your threshold drops.

The week of blank journal pages begins with the Metabolic Strength Circuit Workout, which gives you plenty of room to record the number of repetitions you perform, what amount of weight you used, and any modifications you may have made to the moves (those described in the exercise instructions or your own). Don't forget to mark how many circuits you complete using the check boxes at the bottom of the page.

Next you'll see the Fat-Burning Cardio Intervals chart, which summarizes your cardio workouts for the week and gives you space to record the date, what type of cardio activity you did, the duration of your exercise, your rate of perceived exertion, and (optionally) your heart rate during both work and recovery intervals.

After each workout, fill out the Weekly Activity EFI Scores chart located on page 340. At the end of the week, you will be able to look back at this page to review your feelings about exercising and about yourself.

Then you'll find enough Food Log pages for 7 days. Each Food Log gives you plenty of room to track what you're eating and drinking and when, as well as an at-a-glance summation of how you did each day in meeting your nutritional goals.

Finally, the week ends with a Weekly Measurements sheet. Here you can jot down your weight and the circumference of your chest, waist, hips, thighs, and biceps to keep track of how many pounds and inches you're losing. All you need are a bathroom scale and a measuring tape. (It can be helpful if you have a partner do this for you.) You'll also have room to record any observations or additional notes at the bottom of the page.

If you are also tracking your blood pressure, blood glucose, and other metrics, remember to make an appointment with your doctor every 12 weeks or so. You can fill in your updated numbers in the Starting Stats chart on page 330.

Beginning on page 331, you'll see sample journal pages all filled out—you don't have to complete your pages exactly like this, though. Ultimately, this journal is your weight-loss tool, so use it in whatever way works best for you!

STARTING STATS

Calculating BMI. Use the following formula: Multiply your weight in pounds by 703. Divide that number by your height in inches. Divide that number by your height in inches again. Or skip the math and use the BMI calculator at www.prevention.com/bmi for individualized results.

Taking your measurements. It can be difficult to measure yourself accurately, so ask a partner to help you out if you can. Measure your chest at the fullest part (for women, around the bust). Your waist should be measured approximately 2 inches above your navel, around the narrowest part of your middle. Take your hip measurement around the widest part. For thighs and biceps, measure the fullest part on each limb, keeping your muscles relaxed.

VT1: After you've taken the VT1 test described in Chapter 5, note the results below.

Resting heart rate and bloodwork. This is optional. If you want to check your progress, ask your doctor for the medical tests listed below. Repeat after 12 weeks or more.

DATE/TIME: _____

Weight: _____   Body mass index (BMI): _____

INCHES: Chest: _____   Left thigh: _____   Right thigh: _____

Waist: _____   Left biceps: _____   Right biceps: _____

Hips: _____

VT1: Speed (mph)/incline (%): _____   RPE (1–10): _____   Heart rate: _____

Bloodwork (optional)

	PROGRAM START DATE: _____	AFTER 12 WEEKS DATE: _____
Resting heart rate		
Systolic blood pressure		
Diastolic blood pressure		
Triglycerides		
Total cholesterol		
HDL cholesterol		
LDL cholesterol		
Glucose		
Other		

Metabolic Strength Circuit Workout

MOVE	WORKOUT 1 DAY/DATE: *Monday, 5/7*	WORKOUT 2 DAY/DATE: *Wednesday, 5/9*
Romanian deadlift	Reps: *12* Weight: *8 lb* Notes:	Reps: *13* Weight: *8 lb* Notes:
Chest press	Reps: *8* Weight: *8 lb* Notes:	Reps: *10* Weight: *8 lb* Notes:
Bent-over row	Reps: *10* Weight: *8 lb* Notes:	Reps: *11* Weight: *5 lb* Notes:
Dumbbell squat	Reps: *12* Weight: *0* Notes: *no weights*	Reps: *12* Weight: *5 lb* Notes:
Standing shoulder press	Reps: *10* Weight: *5 lb* Notes:	Reps: *11* Weight: *5 lb* Notes:
Stationary lunge	Reps: *12* Weight: *8 lb* Notes:	Reps: *12* Weight: *8 lb* Notes:
Triceps press	Reps: *10* Weight: *5 lb* Notes:	Reps: *10* Weight: *5 lb* Notes:
Biceps curl	Reps: *10* Weight: *5 lb* Notes:	Reps: *12* Weight: *5 lb* Notes:
Plié squat	Reps: *12* Weight: *8 lb* Notes:	Reps: *13* Weight: *8 lb* Notes:
Pushup	Reps: *12* Weight: Notes: *knees on floor*	Reps: *10* Weight: Notes:
Plank	Reps: *12* Weight: *8 lb* Notes: *started at full pushup position — hold 30 sec.*	Reps: *12* Weight: *8 lb* Notes: *hold 20 sec.*
Bicycle	Reps: *11* Weight: Notes:	Reps: *12* Weight: Notes:
CIRCUITS COMPLETED	1 ⊗ 2 ⊗ 3 ◯	1 ⊗ 2 ⊗ 3 ⊗

Use the notes field to record any modifications or hold times for each exercise.

Fat-Burning Cardio Intervals

MINUTES	EFFORT	TALK TEST	HEART RATE (OPTIONAL)	RPE
0–3	Light (warmup)	Easy conversation	120	3–4
3–6	Medium-high	Challenging (short phrases)	150	7
6–10	Medium	Easier (short sentences)	140	5
10–13	Medium-high	Challenging	150	7
13–17	Medium	Easier	140	5
17–20	Medium-high	Challenging	150	7
20–24	Medium	Easier	140	5
24–25	Light (cooldown)	Easy	120	3–4

WORKOUT 1	WORKOUT 2	WORKOUT 3 (OPTIONAL)
Date: 5/8	Date: 5/10	Date: 5/12
Activity: treadmill	Activity: treadmill	Activity: swimming
Length: 1 hr.	Length: 1 hr.	Length: 30 min.
Work RPE: 7	Work RPE: 7	Work RPE: 5
Recovery RPE: 4	Recovery RPE: 4	Recovery RPE: 3

Weekly Activity EFI Scores

Score each emotion according to how strongly you feel it after every workout, using the scale below.

0 = Do not feel .... **1** = Feel slightly .... **2** = Feel moderately
3 = Feel strongly .... **4** = Feel very strongly

	STRENGTH WORKOUT 1	STRENGTH WORKOUT 2	CARDIO WORKOUT 1	CARDIO WORKOUT 2	CARDIO WORKOUT 3
Day/Date	5/7	5/9	5/8	5/10	5/12
1. Refreshed	1	2	1	2	3
2. Calm	1	2	2	3	3
3. Fatigued	3	3	2	2	2
4. Enthusiastic	1	2	3	3	4
5. Relaxed	2	2	2	2	2
6. Energetic	1	1	2	2	3
7. Happy	2	2	2	3	4
8. Tired	3	3	2	2	2
9. Revived	2	2	2	3	3
10. Peaceful	1	1	2	2	2
11. Worn-out	3	2	1	2	1
12. Upbeat	2	1	3	4	4
	TOTALS				
Positive engagement (4, 7, 12)	5	5	8	10	12
Revitalization (1, 6, 9)	4	5	5	7	9
Tranquility (2, 5, 10)	4	5	6	7	7
Physical exhaustion (3, 8, 11)	9	8	5	6	5

⟳ Food Log

If you're eating according to our meal plan, you don't need to track much more than calories and fiber intake, because our meals and snacks are designed for a healthy diet. But if you're making your own food choices or following doctor-prescribed dietary restrictions, you may want to watch other nutritional elements such as saturated fat, sodium, protein, and carbs. The Food Log is flexible so that you can fill in as much or as little information as you need to help you stay on track.

Week _1_ **Day 2**   **Date:** _5/8_

	FOOD/DRINKS	TIME	CALORIES	FIBER (GRAMS)
Breakfast	Take-Along Egg Wrap, water	8 a.m.	308	11
Lunch	Taco Salad, water	12:30 pm.	444	13
Dinner	BK Veggie Burger, side salad, no dressing, water	6 pm.	450	8
Snack 1	1 cup cooked edamame beans, no shells, green tea	3 pm.	244	10
Snack 2	Yogurt with banana and mini M&M's	8:30 pm.	190	3
(Optional) Snack 3	None			

DAILY NUTRITIONAL TOTALS

Calories: _1,636_   Fiber: _45_ g   Sat. fat: _3.5_ g

Protein: ____ g   Carbs: ____ g   Sodium: ____ mg

Water: ⊗ ⊗ ⊗ ⊗ ⊗ ⊗ ○ ○ ○ ○

Weekly Measurements

DATE/TIME: *May 12, 2011*

Weight: *154 lb*   Body Mass Index (BMI): *26*

INCHES: Chest: *33*   Left thigh: *$20^1/_4$*   Right thigh: *$20^1/_2$*

Waist: *35*   Left biceps: *$8^1/_2$*   Right biceps: *$8^3/_4$*

Hips: *38*

ADDITIONAL OBSERVATIONS: *I feel really good about getting through a whole week of exercising. I followed the meal plan pretty well, though choosing my own snacks and meals seems to result in exceeding my calorie goals for the day. Next week I'm going to spend more time planning so I can use the recipes included in the book. I'm sleeping better at night and feel like I have more energy during the day, which is awesome!*

Metabolic Strength Circuit Workout

Use the chart below to create your own series of moves. You can repeat those listed in any of the prestructured weeks of the program or choose from the list on page 306. If you're repeating the program, add an extra challenge by doing more reps, using heavier weights, adding modifications, or even adding another circuit to your session (three is your maximum—you don't want to overdo it). If you're customizing, choose moves that exercise all seven primary body regions: chest, arms, shoulders, back, legs, butt, and core. Rest about 15 seconds between moves and a full 60 seconds at the end of the circuit. Do this workout two or three times this week on nonconsecutive days.

What you'll need: Light and medium weights; a sturdy chair or bench; and a mat (optional).

Use the notes field to record any modifications or hold times for each exercise.

MOVE	WORKOUT 1 DAY/DATE: _____	WORKOUT 2 DAY/DATE: _____
	Reps: _____ Weight: _____ Notes: _____	Reps: _____ Weight: _____ Notes: _____
	Reps: _____ Weight: _____ Notes: _____	Reps: _____ Weight: _____ Notes: _____
	Reps: _____ Weight: _____ Notes: _____	Reps: _____ Weight: _____ Notes: _____
	Reps: _____ Weight: _____ Notes: _____	Reps: _____ Weight: _____ Notes: _____
	Reps: _____ Weight: _____ Notes: _____	Reps: _____ Weight: _____ Notes: _____
	Reps: _____ Weight: _____ Notes: _____	Reps: _____ Weight: _____ Notes: _____
	Reps: _____ Weight: _____ Notes: _____	Reps: _____ Weight: _____ Notes: _____

MOVE	WORKOUT 1 DAY/DATE: _____		WORKOUT 2 DAY/DATE: _____	
	Reps: _____ Weight: _____ Notes: _____ _____		Reps: _____ Weight: _____ Notes: _____ _____	
	Reps: _____ Weight: _____ Notes: _____ _____		Reps: _____ Weight: _____ Notes: _____ _____	
	Reps: _____ Weight: _____ Notes: _____ _____		Reps: _____ Weight: _____ Notes: _____ _____	
	Reps: _____ Weight: _____ Notes: _____ _____		Reps: _____ Weight: _____ Notes: _____ _____	
	Reps: _____ Weight: _____ Notes: _____ _____		Reps: _____ Weight: _____ Notes: _____ _____	
	Reps: _____ Weight: _____ Notes: _____ _____		Reps: _____ Weight: _____ Notes: _____ _____	
	Reps: _____ Weight: _____ Notes: _____ _____		Reps: _____ Weight: _____ Notes: _____ _____	
	Reps: _____ Weight: _____ Notes: _____ _____		Reps: _____ Weight: _____ Notes: _____ _____	
	Reps: _____ Weight: _____ Notes: _____ _____		Reps: _____ Weight: _____ Notes: _____ _____	
	Reps: _____ Weight: _____ Notes: _____ _____		Reps: _____ Weight: _____ Notes: _____ _____	
	Reps: _____ Weight: _____ Notes: _____ _____		Reps: _____ Weight: _____ Notes: _____ _____	
	Reps: _____ Weight: _____ Notes: _____ _____		Reps: _____ Weight: _____ Notes: _____ _____	
CIRCUITS COMPLETED	1 ○ 2 ○ 3 ○		1 ○ 2 ○ 3 ○	

Fat-Burning Cardio Intervals

Use the chart below to write in your interval routine. If you're repeating the intervals from the program, customize by adding more work/rest combos, extending your warmups and cooldowns, or shifting your work-to-recovery ratios. Do your intervals two or three times a week; if you're doing steady-state cardio, try to structure your steady-state workouts so that you're doing a total of 150 minutes a week, either five times at a moderate intensity or three times at a vigorous effort.

You can combine a number of interval and steady-state workouts for the week however you choose.

What you'll need: You can do any form of steady-state cardio, but for best results with intervals, try to stick with the same type of workout that you did for your VT1 test.

MINUTES	EFFORT	TALK TEST	HEART RATE (OPTIONAL)	RPE

MINUTES	EFFORT	TALK TEST	HEART RATE (OPTIONAL)	RPE

WORKOUT 1	WORKOUT 2	WORKOUT 3 (OPTIONAL)
Date:	Date:	Date:
Activity:	Activity:	Activity:
Length:	Length:	Length:
Work RPE:	Work RPE:	Work RPE:
Recovery RPE:	Recovery RPE:	Recovery RPE:

WORKOUT 4 (OPTIONAL)	WORKOUT 5 (OPTIONAL)	NOTES
Date:	Date:	
Activity:	Activity:	
Length:	Length:	
Work RPE:	Work RPE:	
Recovery RPE:	Recovery RPE:	

Weekly Activity EFI Scores

Score each emotion according to how strongly you feel it after every workout, using the scale below.

0 = Do not feel ⋯⋯⋯ **1** = Feel slightly ⋯⋯⋯ **2** = Feel moderately

3 = Feel strongly ⋯⋯⋯ **4** = Feel very strongly

	STRENGTH WORKOUT 1	STRENGTH WORKOUT 2	CARDIO WORKOUT 1	CARDIO WORKOUT 2	CARDIO WORKOUT 3
Day/Date					
1. Refreshed					
2. Calm					
3. Fatigued					
4. Enthusiastic					
5. Relaxed					
6. Energetic					
7. Happy					
8. Tired					
9. Revived					
10. Peaceful					
11. Worn-out					
12. Upbeat					
TOTALS					
Positive engagement (4, 7, 12)					
Revitalization (1, 6, 9)					
Tranquility (2, 5, 10)					
Physical exhaustion (3, 8, 11)					

↻ Food Log

Week _____ Day 1   Date: _____

	FOOD/DRINKS	TIME	CALORIES	FIBER (GRAMS)
Breakfast				
Lunch				
Dinner				
Snack 1				
Snack 2				
(Optional) Snack 3				

DAILY NUTRITIONAL TOTALS			
	Calories: _____	Fiber: _____ g	Sat. fat: _____ g
	Protein: _____ g	Carbs: _____ g	Sodium: _____ mg
	Water: ○ ○ ○ ○ ○ ○ ○ ○ ○ ○		

Food Log

Week _____ Day 2   Date: _____

	FOOD/DRINKS	TIME	CALORIES	FIBER (GRAMS)
Breakfast				
Lunch				
Dinner				
Snack 1				
Snack 2				
(Optional) Snack 3				

DAILY NUTRITIONAL TOTALS	Calories: _____	Fiber: _____ g	Sat. fat: _____ g
	Protein: _____ g	Carbs: _____ g	Sodium: _____ mg
	Water: ○ ○ ○ ○ ○ ○ ○ ○ ○ ○		

Food Log

Week _____ Day 3   Date: _____

	FOOD/DRINKS	TIME	CALORIES	FIBER (GRAMS)
Breakfast				
Lunch				
Dinner				
Snack 1				
Snack 2				
(Optional) Snack 3				

DAILY NUTRITIONAL TOTALS

Calories: _____   Fiber: _____ g   Sat. fat: _____ g

Protein: _____ g   Carbs: _____ g   Sodium: _____ mg

Water: ○ ○ ○ ○ ○ ○ ○ ○ ○ ○

Food Log

Week _____ **Day 4**   **Date:** _____

	FOOD/DRINKS	TIME	CALORIES	FIBER (GRAMS)
Breakfast				
Lunch				
Dinner				
Snack 1				
Snack 2				
(Optional) Snack 3				

DAILY NUTRITIONAL TOTALS			
	Calories: _____	Fiber: _____ g	Sat. fat: _____ g
	Protein: _____ g	Carbs: _____ g	Sodium: _____ mg
	Water: ○ ○ ○ ○ ○ ○ ○ ○ ○ ○		

Food Log

Week _____ Day 5   Date: _____

	FOOD/DRINKS	TIME	CALORIES	FIBER (GRAMS)
Breakfast				
Lunch				
Dinner				
Snack 1				
Snack 2				
(Optional) Snack 3				

DAILY NUTRITIONAL TOTALS

Calories: _____   Fiber: _____ g   Sat. fat: _____ g

Protein: _____ g   Carbs: _____ g   Sodium: _____ mg

Water: ○ ○ ○ ○ ○ ○ ○ ○ ○ ○

Food Log

Week _____ Day 6   Date:_____

	FOOD/DRINKS	TIME	CALORIES	FIBER (GRAMS)
Breakfast				
Lunch				
Dinner				
Snack 1				
Snack 2				
(Optional) Snack 3				

DAILY NUTRITIONAL TOTALS

Calories: _____   Fiber: _____ g   Sat. fat: _____ g

Protein: _____ g   Carbs: _____ g   Sodium: _____ mg

Water: ○ ○ ○ ○ ○ ○ ○ ○ ○ ○

Food Log

Week _____ Day 7   Date: _____

	FOOD/DRINKS	TIME	CALORIES	FIBER (GRAMS)
Breakfast				
Lunch				
Dinner				
Snack 1				
Snack 2				
(Optional) Snack 3				

DAILY NUTRITIONAL TOTALS

Calories: _____   Fiber: _____ g   Sat. fat: _____ g

Protein: _____ g   Carbs: _____ g   Sodium: _____ mg

Water: ○ ○ ○ ○ ○ ○ ○ ○ ○ ○

Weekly Measurements

DATE/TIME: _____

        Weight: _____   Body mass index (BMI): _____

INCHES: Chest: _____   Left thigh: _____   Right thigh: _____

        Waist: _____   Left biceps: _____   Right biceps: _____

        Hips: _____

ADDITIONAL OBSERVATIONS: _____

_____

_____

_____

_____

_____

_____

_____

_____

_____

_____

_____

_____

_____

_____

_____

Endnotes

PART I

1. Natalie Digate Muth, "What Are the Guidelines for Percentage of Body Fat Loss?" www.acefitness.org (accessed November 10, 2010).

2. Duke University Medical Center, "Physical Inactivity Rapidly Increases Visceral Fat; Exercise Can Reverse Accumulation," *Science Daily,* May 29, 2003, www.sciencedaily.com (accessed November 13, 2010).

3. Richard Cotton, ed., *Personal Trainer Manual,* 2nd ed. (San Diego: American Council on Exercise, 1996): 7.

4. Xuemei Sui and others, "Cardiorespiratory Fitness and Adiposity as Mortality Predictors in Older Adults," *Journal of the American Medical Association* 298, no. 21 (December 5, 2007): 2507–16.

5. Christian Werner and others, "Physical Exercise Prevents Cellular Senescence in Circulating Leukocytes and in the Vessel Wall," *Circulation* 120, no. 24 (December 15, 2009): 2438–47.

6. Joseph E. Donnelly and others, "Appropriate Physical Activity Intervention Strategies for Weight Loss and Prevention of Weight Regain for Adults," *Medicine and Science in Sports and Exercise* 41, no. 2 (February 2009): 459–71.

7. "NWCR Facts," www.nwcr.ws/Research (accessed November 13, 2010).

8. P. J. Arciero and others, "Increased Dietary Protein and Combined High Intensity Aerobic and Resistance Exercise Improves Body Fat Distribution and Cardiovascular Risk Factors," *International Journal of Sports Nutrition and Exercise Metabolism* 4, no. 16 (August 16, 2006): 373–92.

9. Len Kravitz, "Fat Facts," www.unm.edu/~lkravitz (accessed November 13, 2010).

10. G. J. Bell and others, "A Comparison of Fitness Training to a Pedometer-Based Walking Program Matched for Total Energy Cost," *Journal of Physical Activity and Health* 2, no. 7 (March 7, 2010): 203–13.

11. A. Stasiulis and others, "Aerobic Exercise-Induced Changes in Body Composition and Blood Lipids in Young Women," *Medicina (Kaunas)* 46, no. 2 (2010): 129–34.

12. "Q&A," www.acefitness.org/fitnessqanda (accessed November 16, 2010).

13. Gary R. Hunter and others, "Resistance Training Increases Total Energy Expenditure and Free-Living Physical Activity in Older Adults," *Journal of Applied Physiology* 89, no. 3 (September 2000): 977–84.

14. G. R. Hunter and others, "Resistance Training Conserves Fat-Free Mass and Resting Energy Expenditure Following Weight Loss," *Obesity* 16, no. 5 (May 2008): 1045–51.

15. Andrew Hill, "Does Dieting Make You Fat?" *British Journal of Nutrition* 92, supplement 1 (2004): S15–S18.

16. Michael J. Ormsbee and others, "Fat Metabolism and Acute Resistance Exercise in Trained Men," *Journal of Applied Physiology* 102, no. 5 (May 2007): 1767–72.

17. Wayne Westcott, *Strength Fitness: Physiological Principles and Training Techniques,* 2nd edition (Dubuque, IA: William C. Brown, 1991): 74–75.

18. W. J. Kraemer and others, "Influence of Exercise Training on Physiological and Performance Changes with Weight Loss in Men," *Medicine and Science in Sports and Exercise* 31, no. 9 (September 1999): 1320–29.

19. B. E. Ainsworth, "The Compendium of Physical Activities Tracking Guide," January 2002, prevention.sph.sc.edu/tools/docs/documents_compendium.pdf (accessed November 16, 2010).

20. Ibid.

21. C. B. Scott and others, "Aerobic, Anaerobic, and Excess Postexercise Oxygen Consumption Energy Expenditure of Muscular Endurance and Strength: 1-Set of Bench Press to Muscular Fatigue," *Journal of Strength Conditioning Research* (August 10, 2010).

22. W. J. Kraemer and others, "Resistance Training Combined with Bench-Step Aerobics Enhances Women's Health Profile," *Medicine & Science in Sports & Exercise* 33, no. 2 (February 2001): 259–269.

23. M. D. Schuenke, R. P. Mikat, and J. M. McBride, "Effect of an Acute Period of Resistance Exercise on Excess Postexercise Oxygen Consumption: Implications for Body Mass Management," *European Journal of Applied Physiology* 86, no. 6 (March 2002): 411–17.

24. M. R. Rhea and others, "A Comparison of Linear and Daily Undulating Periodized Programs with Equated Volume and Intensity for Strength," *Journal of Strength and Conditioning Research* 16, no. 2 (May 2002): 250–55.

25. Said Ahmaidi and others, "Effects of Interval Training at the Ventilatory Threshold on Clinical and Cardiorespiratory Responses in Elderly Humans," *European Journal of Applied Physiology and Occupational Physiology* 78, no. 2 (July 1998): 170–76.

26. New Leaf Technologies, white paper provided to author, 2010.

27. N. A. Burd and others, "Low-Load High Volume Resistance Exercise Stimulates Muscle Protein Synthesis More Than High-Load Low Volume Resistance Exercise in Young Men," *PLoS OnE* 5, no. 8 (August 9, 2010): e12033.

28. E. D. Rose and G. Parfitt, "Exercise Experience Influences Affective and Motivational Outcomes of Prescribed and Self-Selected Intensity Exercise," *Scandinavian Journal of Medicine and Science in Sports* (July 6, 2010).

29. J. Achten and A. E. Jeukendrup, "Optimizing Fat Oxidation through Exercise and Diet," *Nutrition* 20, no. 7–8 (July–August 2004): 716–27.

30. Lisa M. Nackers, Kathryn M. Ross, and Michael G. Perri, "The Association between Rate of Initial Weight Loss and Long-Term Success in Obesity Treatment: Does Slow and Steady Win the Race?" *International Journal of Behavioral Medicine* 17, no. 3 (September 2010): 161–7.

31. Gary R. Hunter and others, "Exercise Training Prevents Regain of Visceral Fat for 1 Year Following Weight Loss," *Obesity* 18, no. 4 (2010): 690–95.

PART II

1. Christopher D. Black and others, "Ginger (*Zingiber officinale*) Reduces Muscle Pain Caused by Eccentric Exercise," *Journal of Pain* 1, no. 9 (September 2010): 894–903.

2. Daniel Pereles and others, "A Large, Randomized, Prospective Study of the Impact of a Pre-Run Stretch on the Risk of Injury in Teenage and Older Runners," www.usatf.org/stretchstudy/protocol.asp (accessed November 16, 2010).

3. C. H. Chen and others, "Effects of Flexibility Training on Eccentric Exercise-Induced Muscle Damage," *Medicine and Science in Sports and Exercise* (August 2, 2010).

4. T. Yamaguchi and K. Ishii, "Effects of Static Stretching for 30 seconds and Dynamic Stretching on Leg Extension Power," *Journal of Strength and Conditioning Research* 19, no. 3 (August 2005): 677–83.

5. T. Little and A. G. Williams, "Effects of Differential Stretching Protocols during Warm-Ups on High-Speed Motor Capacities in Professional Soccer Players," *Journal of Strength and Conditioning Research* 20, no. 1 (February 2006): 203–7.

6. "How Much Physical Activity Do Adults Need?" www.cdc.gov/physicalactivity (accessed November 16, 2010).

7. "Dietary Reference Intakes: Water, Potassium, Sodium, Chloride, and Sulfate," www.iom.edu/Reports/2004/Dietary-Reference-Intakes-Water-Potassium-Sodium-Chloride-and-Sulfate.aspx (accessed November 16, 2010).

8. Michael Boschmann and others, "Water-Induced Thermogenesis," *Journal of Clinical Endocrinology & Metabolism* 88, no. 12 (December 2003): 6015–19.

9. "NWCR Facts," www.nwcr.ws/research (accessed November 13, 2010).

10. D. Benardot and others, "Between-Meal Energy Intake Effects on Body Composition, Performance, and Total Caloric Consumption in Athletes," *Medicine and Science in Sports and Exercise* 37, no. 5 (May 2005): S339.

PART III

1. S. Li and others, "Physical Activity Attenuates the Genetic Predisposition to Obesity in 20,000 Men and Women from EPIC-Norfolk Prospective Population Study," *PLoS Medicine* 7, no. 8 (August 31, 2010): e1000332.

2. G. N. Healy and others, "Objectively Measured Sedentary Time, Physical Activity, and Metabolic Risk: The Australian Diabetes, Obesity, and Lifestyle Study (Aus-Diab)," *Diabetes Care* 31, no. 2 (February 2008): 369–71.

3. F. B. Hu and others, "Television Watching and Other Sedentary Behaviors in Relation to Risk of Obesity and Type 2 Diabetes Mellitus in Women," *Journal of the American Medical Association* 289, no. 14 (April 2003): 1785–91.

4. A. V. Nedeltcheva, "Insufficient Sleep Undermines Dietary Efforts to Reduce Adiposity," *Annals of Internal Medicine* 153, no. 7 (October 5, 2010): 435–41.

5. C. A. Shively, T. C. Register, and T. B. Clarkson, "Social Stress, Visceral Obesity, and Coronary Artery Atherosclerosis: Product of a Primate Adaptation," *American Journal of Primatology* 71, no. 9 (September 2009): 742–51.

6. Kathleen J. Melanson, Kaitlyn E. Reti, and Daniel L. Kresge, "Impact of Chewing Gum on Appetite, Meal Intake, and Mood under Controlled Conditions," *Obesity* 2009, Washington D.C., October 2009.

7. C. H. Gilhooly and others, "Food Cravings and Energy Regulation: The Characteristics of Craved Foods and Their Relationship with Eating Behaviors and Weight Change during 6 Months of Dietary Energy Restriction," *International Journal of Obesity,* Advance Electronic version (June 26, 2007).

8. Denise Benitez and others, "Yoga Practice Is Associated with Attenuated Weight Gain in Healthy, Middle-Aged Men and Women," *Alternative Therapies in Health and Medicine* 11, no. 4 (July–August 2005): 28–33.

PART IV

1. Jeong In Joo and others, "Proteomic Analysis for Antiobesity Potential of Capsaicin on White Adipose Tissue in Rats Fed with a High Fat Diet," *Journal of Proteome Research* 9, no. 6 (June 4, 2010): 2977–87.

2. K. L. Funk and others, "Associations of Internet Website Use with Weight Change in a Long-Term Weight Loss Maintenance Program," *Journal of Medical Internet Research* 12, no. 3 (July 27, 2010): e29.

3. Judy McBride, "Cinnamon Extract Boosts Insulin Sensitivity," *Agricultural Research* 48, no. 7 (July 2000): 21.

4. M. A. Wien, "Almonds vs. Complex Carbohydrates in a Weight Reduction Program," *International Journal of Obesity Related Metabolic Disorders* 27, no. 11 (November 2003): 1365–72.

5. M. Schulz and others, "Identification of a Food Pattern Characterized by High-Fiber and Low-Fat Food Choices Associated with Low Prospective Weight Change in the EPIC-Potsdam Cohort," *Journal of Nutrition* 135, no. 5 (May 2005): 1183–9.

6. N. M. McKeown and others, "Whole- and Refined-Grain Intakes Are Differentially

Associated with Abdominal Visceral and Subcutaneous Adiposity in Healthy Adults: The Framingham Heart Study," *American Journal of Clinical Nutrition* 92, no. 5 (November 2010): 1165–71.

7. "Dietary Reference Intakes: Macronutrients," www.iom.edu/Reports/2004/C5GD2DD7840544979A549EC47E56A02B.ashx (accessed November 16, 2010).

8. "Dietary Supplement Fact Sheet," ods.od.nih.gov/factsheets/magnesium/#h3 (accessed November 16, 2010).

9. R. Lopez-Ridaura and others, "Magnesium Intake and Risk of Type 2 Diabetes in Men and Women," *Diabetes Care* 27 (January 2004): 270–1.

10. D. Mozaffarian and others, "Trans Fatty Acids and Cardiovascular Disease," *New England Journal of Medicine* 354, no. 15 (April 13, 2006): 1601–13.

11. F. B. Hu, J. E. Manson, and W. C. Willett, "Types of Dietary Fat and Risk of Coronary Heart Disease: A Critical Review," *Journal of the American College of Nutrition* 20 (February 2001): 5–19.

12. I. Thorsdottir and others, "Randomized Trial of Weight-Loss Diets for Young Adults Varying in Fish and Fish Oil Content," *International Journal of Obesity* 10 (October 31, 2007): 1560–66.

13. E. A. Dennis and others, "Water Consumption Increases Weight Loss during a Hypocaloric Diet Intervention in Middle-Aged and Older Adults," *Obesity* 18, no. 2 (February 2010): 300–7.

14. K. C. Maki and others, "Green Tea Catechin Consumption Enhances Exercise-Induced Abdominal Fat Loss in Overweight and Obese Adults," *Journal of Nutrition* 139, no. 2 (February 2009): 264–70.

15. S. Uchiyama and others, "Prevention of Diet-Induced Obesity by Dietary Black Tea Polyphenols Extract in Vitro and in Vivo," *Nutrition* (June 2, 2010).

16. E. Lopez-Garcia and others, "The Relationship of Coffee Consumption with Mortality," *Annals of Internal Medicine* 148 (June 17, 2008): 1–40.

17. J. S. Vander Wal and others, "Egg Breakfast Enhances Weight Loss," *International Journal of Obesity* 32, no. 10 (October 2008): 1545–51.

18. "Cutting Salt, Improving Health," www.nyc.gov/html/doh/html/cardio/cardio-salt-initiative.shtml (accessed November 17, 2010).

19. "Physical Activity and Public Health Guidelines." www.acsm.org (accessed November 17, 2010).

20. A. A. Gorin and others, "Promoting Long-Term Weight Control: Does Dieting Consistency Matter?," *International Journal of Obesity Related Metabolic Disorders* 29, no. 1 (February 2004): 278–81.

21. "NWCR Facts," www.nwcr.ws/Research (accessed November 17, 2010).

22. M. S. Buchowski and others, "Physical Activity and Obesity Gap between Black and White Women in the Southeastern U.S," *American Journal of Preventive Medicine* 39, no. 2 (August 2010): 140–7.

23. F. B. Hu and others, "Television Watching and Other Sedentary Behaviors in Relation to Risk of Obesity and Type 2 Diabetes Mellitus in Women," *Journal of the American Medical Association* 289, no. 14 (April 9, 2003): 1785–91.

24. Ibid.

25. Ibid.

26. "Physical Inactivity Rapidly Increases Visceral Fat; Exercise Can Reverse Accumulation," www.dukehealth.org (accessed November 17, 2010).

27. Jean-Philippe Chaput and others, "The Association between Sleep Duration and Weight Gain in Adults: A 6-Year Prospective Study from the Quebec Family Study," *Sleep* 31, no. 4 (April 1, 2008): 517–523.

28. Funk and others, "Associations of Internet Website Use with Weight Change in a Long-Term Weight Loss Maintenance Program," *Journal of Medical Internet Research* 12, no. 3 (July 27, 2010): e29.

29. L. D. Frank, M. A. Andresen, and T. L. Schmid, "Obesity Relationships with Community Design, Physical Activity, and Time Spent in Cars," *American Journal of Preventive Medicine* 27, no. 2 (August 2004): 87–96.

Index

Underscored page references indicate sidebars. **Boldface** references indicate photographs.

Dips *(cont.)*
    Vegetables with Almond Butter Dipping
        Sauce, 273
    Zesty Roasted Red Pepper Dip, 274
Doctor approval, of exercise, 15
Dumbbell squat, 103, **103**
Dunkin Donuts, 232
Duren, Burt, 52–53, **52**, **53**
Dynamic stretching
    benefits of, 43
    in on-board program, 56, 57–62, **58–62**
    for strength training, 98, 99, 118, 136
Dynamic warmup, for week 4, 156
    around-the-clock lunges, 159, **159**
    bodyweight squat and arm reach, 158,
        158
    cat back/down dog, 157, **157**

E

Eating out. *See* Restaurant meals
Eating plan. *See* Turn Up Your Fat Burn
        Eating Plan
Edamame
    Fiery Edamame, 212
    Flank Steak with Edamame, Black
        Pepper, and Green Onions, 267
Eggs
    Egg Sandwich, 207
    Italian Omelet, 244
    Red Hot Eggs, 243
    Take-Along Egg Wrap, 207
    Veggie Scrambled Eggs and Crackers,
        207
    for weight loss, 200
Elastic tubing, 305
Emotional eating, 150
Emotional response to exercise,
        monitoring, 91–92, 93
Energy bars, 191, 217
EPOC (excess postoxygen consumption), 21
Equipment
    for metabolic strength circuit, 98, 119,
        137, 160
    for on-board strength workout, 63
    for Turn Up Your Fat Burn program,
        46–48
    weights (*see* Weights)
Espresso
    Cappuccino Freeze, 289
    Espresso Parfait, 288

Excuses for not exercising, 113
Exercise. *See also specific exercises and
        workouts*
    aerobic (*see* Aerobic exercise)
    continuing, after 4-week plan, 294
    doctor approval of, 15
    excuses for skipping, 113
    for fat loss, 4, 5–6, 9, 10, 11, 14, 19, 26, 28,
        29, 325
    health benefits of, 7, 8
    inadequate results from, 7–8
        mistakes contributing to, 8–10
    minimum requirements for, 295–96
    monitoring emotional response to,
        91–92, 93
    for weight maintenance, 7, 325, 326
Exercise-Induced Feeling Inventory
        (EFI), 91–92, 93
Exercise intensity, methods of
        determining, 82–86
Exercise rut, 8

F

Fat, body
    alternate ways of reducing, 131
    average percentage of, 4
    burning or losing, 29
    excess of, 3, 4
    exercise for burning or losing, 4, 5–6, 9,
        10, 11, 14, 19, 26, 28, 29, 325
    functions of, 3
    triglycerides in, 5
    types of, 4
    VT1 for burning, 11, 12, 13, 25, 82, 83
Fats, dietary
    for building your own meal, 223–24
    functions of, 4, 185
    good vs. bad types of, 195–98
    for preventing cravings, 150
    triglycerides in, 5
Fatty acids, 5, 6, 11. *See also* Omega-3 fatty
        acids; Omega-6 fatty acids
Fiber
    benefits of, 190–92
    in Build Your Own Meal chart,
        222–23
    foods high in, 205
    recommended intake of, 190, 192, 200,
        204, 226
    soluble vs. insoluble, 193

Muscle (*cont.*)
    effect on metabolism, 9, 13, 14, 15
    exercise variety and, 22
    metabolic circuit workouts toning, 21–22
    strength training increasing, 9, 15
Muscle loss, causes of, 9, 14
Muscle soreness, from strength training, 38–40, 42, 57, <u>57</u>
Mustard
    Dijon Grilled Chicken, 266
My Health Trackers tool, 188, 326
MyPyramidTracker.gov, 188

N

National Weight Control Registry, 7, 50, 322–23
Nonlinear periodization, 22
Nuts
    Almondy Apple, 219
    benefits of, <u>189</u>
    Biscotti and Almonds, 220
    Brown Rice and Cashew Salad, 257
    Cashew Couscous, 212
    Cashews and Peaches, 219
    Chicken Amandine and Lemon Peas, 214
    Couscous with Tomatoes, Chickpeas, and Brazil Nuts, 212–13
    Crackers with Walnut-Date Salad, 218
    Cream Cheese Crackers with Cinnamon-Sugar Peanuts, 221
    Crunchy Pistachio Pie, 291
    Grilled Cheese and Nutty Tomato Soup, 210
    Maple-Pecan Oatmeal, 284
    Maple Walnut Quinoa with Roasted Chicken, 214
    Peanut Cereal Bars, 241
    Pear with Almond Cream, 287
    Pecan Oatmeal, 206
    Pudding and Pecans, 220
    Walnut-Cranberry Biscotti, 292
    Walnuts and Raisins, 220
    White Chocolate, Pecans, and Pretzels, 221

O

Oatmeal
    Maple-Pecan Oatmeal, 284
    Pecan Oatmeal, 206

Obesity
    body mass index indicating, 4
    TV watching and, 324
Omega-3 fatty acids, 39, 196–97, <u>199</u>
Omega-6 fatty acids, 196, 197, <u>199</u>
On-board program
    candidates for, 56–57
    cardio workout in, 76–77
    dynamic stretches in, 56, 57
        butt kicks, 59, **59**
        cat-back stretch, 61, **61**
        chest back stretch, 62, **62**
        Frankenstein walk, 60, **60**
        knee lift, 58, **58**
    purpose of, 55–56
    strength workout in, 56, 63
        bent-over row, 65, **65**
        bodyweight squat, 64, **64**
        bridge, 72, **72**
        plank, 74, **74**
        pushup, 70, **70**
        seated overhead press, 69, **69**
        side lunge, 68, **68**
        standing torso twist, 67, **67**
        static stretches after, 75, <u>75</u>
        step-up and hold, 66, **66**
        swimmer, 71, **71**
        triceps dip, 73, **73**
    warmup in, 56, 57
Onions
    Chicken with Marinated Blueberries and Red Onions, 265
    Flank Steak with Edamame, Black Pepper, and Green Onions, 267
Out and About food guide, 185
    breakfasts, 226–28
    lunches/dinners, 228, 230, 232
Overhead triceps extension, 170, **170**
Overweight, body mass index indicating, 4

P

Pancakes
    Banana Pancakes, 247
    Raspberry Pancakes, 206, 216
Panda Express, 232
Parfait
    Espresso Parfait, 288
Pasta
    Tilapia and Basil Raspberry Pasta, 215

Vegetarian entrées
  Cashew Couscous, 212
  Colorful Chickpea Stew, 213
  Couscous with Tomatoes, Chickpeas,
      and Brazil Nuts, 212–13
  Dill-Topped Veggie Burger with Sweet
      Potato Fries, 212
  Fiery Edamame, 212
Ventilatory Threshold 1. *See* VT1
Ventilatory Threshold 2. *See* VT2
Visceral fat, 4, <u>29</u>, 325
VT1
  boosting, 22, 24, 25, 26, 112, 130, 149, 174
  determining, 81, 82 (*see also* VT1 test)
  for increasing calorie and fat burn,
      10–13, <u>12</u>, 15
  recording, in journal, 328, <u>330</u>
  of regular exercisers, <u>29</u>
  variations in, 86–87
  workout type affecting, 38
VT1 test, 44, 57, 86–90, <u>89</u>, <u>90</u>, 112, <u>112</u>,
      <u>130</u>, <u>149</u>, <u>175</u>, 296–98
VT2, <u>12</u>, 26, 28, 174

W

Waffles
  Chocolate Raspberry Waffle, 220
Wagner, Hans, <u>323</u>
Walking, increasing amount of, <u>131</u>
Warmups
  for cardio workouts, 45, 46
  for on-board program, 57
  for strength training, 98, 99, 118, 136,
      156–59, **157–59**
  for stretching, 43
Water, cold, for muscle soreness, 39
Water drinking
  for muscle soreness, 39–40
  recommended amount of, 49–50, 198
Waverly, Michael, <u>323</u>
Weekend eating, <u>320</u>
Weekly Activity EFI Scores chart, 329,
      <u>333</u>, <u>340</u>
Weekly Measurements sheet, 329, <u>335</u>, <u>348</u>
Weigh-ins, weekly, <u>295</u>, 324
Weight bench, 46
Weight loss
  alternative factors enhancing, <u>131</u>
  calorie burning for, 6–7, 48

eggs for, 200
fiber for, 192
journaling and, 328
rate of, <u>29</u>
role of diet in, 183
spicy foods aiding, <u>187</u>
strength training for, 13–15
tea boosting, 198
workout mistakes preventing, 8–10
Weight maintenance
  breakfast for, 50
  exercise for, 7
  fiber for, 190, 191, 192
  strength training for, 13–15
  tips for, 323–27
  weekend eating and, <u>320</u>
Weights
  choosing, 42, 46, <u>63</u>
  heavy vs. light, <u>29</u>
  for on-board strength workout, 63
  substitutes for, <u>47</u>
Wendy's, 230
Wenrich, Cindy, <u>27</u>, 86, 190, <u>233</u>, **233**
Whole grains, 192, 223, <u>238</u>
Wood chop, 171, **171**
Workout mistakes, 8–10
Workout planning, 37–40, 295–98
Workouts. *See* Cardio workouts; Metabolic
      strength circuits
Work-to-recovery ratios, in interval
      training, 25, **25**, <u>26</u>
Wraps
  Pear Wrap, 208
  Take-Along Egg Wrap, 207

Y

Yoga, for controlling cravings, <u>151</u>
Yoga mat, 47
Yogurt
  Banana Split, 217
  Espresso Parfait, 288
  Fruity Bean Yogurt, 217
  Savory Dip, 280
  Strawberry Yogurt Freeze, 286
  Strawberry Yogurt with Chocolate-
      Covered Raisins, 217
  Yogurt with Banana and M&M's Minis,
      217